MW00445206

Limit of Liability/Disclaimer of Warranty

Neither we nor any third parties provide any warranty or guarantee as to the accuracy, timeliness, performance, completeness or suitability of the information and materials found or offered in this study guide for any particular purpose. You acknowledge that such information and materials may contain inaccuracies or errors and we expressly exclude liability for any such inaccuracies or errors to the fullest extent permitted by law.

About the Exam

The Certified Nursing Assistant exam consists of a written exam and a clinical skills test. The written (oral) exam, also known as the National Nurse Aide Assessment Program (NNAAP), is a two hour exam consisting of 70 questions. Below is an outline of the exam content:

Domain	Percentage

Physical Care Skills
   A. Activities of Daily Living
   1. Hygiene
   2. Dressing and Grooming
   3. Nutrition and Hydration
   4. Elimination
   5. Rest/Sleep/Comfort
	14%

B. Basic Nursing Skills
   1. Infection Control
   2. Safety/Emergency
   3. Therapeutic and Technical Procedures
   4. Data Collection and Reporting
	39%

C. Restorative Skills
   1. Prevention
   2. Self-care/Independence
	8%

Psychosocial Care Skills A. Emotional and Mental Health Needs	11%
B. Spiritual and Cultural Needs	2%
Role of the Nurse Aide A. Communication	8%
B. Client Rights	7%
C. Legal and Ethical Behavior	3%
D. Member of the Healthcare Team	8%

There are 22 skills that are part of the clinical skills test. You will be asked to perform 5 skills that will be randomly selected. The clinical skills test may last anywhere from 30 to 45 minutes. If you leave out a Critical Element Step or do not perform a Critical Element Step properly, you will not pass the skill. Throughout this book, Critical Element Steps will be in bold type. You will also be evaluated on your indirect care skills. Indirect care skills include communicating with the patient, infection control and safety standards, and respecting patient privacy, comfort, and preferences. The clinical skills that may be tested include:

1. Hand hygiene/washing
2. Applying elastic stockings
3. Assisting with use of bedpans
4. Cleaning dentures
5. Provide mouth care
6. Taking the radial pulse
7. Counting respirations
8. Measure and record manual blood pressure
9. Putting on and removing PPE
10. Dress patients who have an affected (weak) arm
11. Feed patients who cannot feed themselves
12. Give modified bed baths
13. Measure and record urinary output
14. Measure and record weight of ambulatory client
15. Perform modified passive range of motion for one knee and one ankle
16. Perform modified passive range of motion for one shoulder
17. Position patients on their side
18. Provide catheter care
19. Provide perineal care for female patients
20. Provide foot care on one foot
21. Transfer patients from bed to wheelchair using a transfer belt
22. Assisting to ambulate using transfer belt

Physical Care Skills

Basic Nursing Skills

Body Positions

Supine: the patient is lying on their back with their face up.
Prone: the patient is lying on their stomach with their face down.
Lateral Position: the patient is lying on their left or right side.
Sim's Position: the same as the lateral position, except the undermost arm is positioned at the resident's back.
Fowler Position: the patient is lying on their back with the upper body elevated at a 45 to 60 degree angle.
Semi-Fowler Position: the same as the Fowler position, except the upper body is elevated at an angle less than 45 degrees.
Orthopneic Position: the patient is sitting upright, bending forward over pillows.

Infection Control (Medical Asepsis)

Pathogens (bacteria, viruses, fungi, and parasites) are disease causing organisms. Many diseases are communicable, or contagious, and one of the duties of a CNA is to prevent the spread of diseases. Diseases spread through direct contact with infected blood, body fluids, and open wounds; it may also spread through inhalation of infected air droplets. Infections may be local or systemic (affects the entire body).

Signs and symptoms of an infection include fever, chills, elevated white blood count, wounds with a strong odor or drainage, redness around a lesion, malaise (general ill feeling), etc. If infections aren't properly treated, it may lead to sepsis. Sepsis is a life-threatening condition that arises when the body's response to infection causes injury to its own tissues and organs.

Below is a list of common infectious diseases:
- Methicillin Resistant Staphylococcus Aureus (MRSA) is a bacterial infection of the skin that can spread to the bloodstream; it's especially prevalent in hospitals and long term care facilities.
- Tuberculosis (TB) is a bacterial infection that mainly affects the lungs.
- Influenza (Flu) is an infectious diseases caused by a virus; symptoms include a high fever, runny nose, sore throat, muscle pains, headache, coughing, and feeling tired.
- Pneumonia is disease that can be caused by a virus or bacteria. It is commonly a complication of the flu and causes inflammation of the air sacs.
- Common cold
- Scabies is a skin infection caused by tiny mites that cause rashes and intense itching.

- Shingles is an infection caused by a virus that attacks a nerve path, causing pain and disability.
- Healthcare workers are at high risk of contracting Hepatitis B (HBV) and Human Immunodeficiency Virus (HIV).

To prevent or reduce the spread of infectious diseases, CNAs must follow infection control guidelines recommended by the Center for Disease Control (CDC).

Hand Hygiene and Washing

- No artificial nails; nails should be trimmed to less than ¼ inch; no nail polish
- Wash hands with soap and hot water for 30 seconds.
- Use hand lotion to prevent dry and cracked skin caused by frequent hand washing.

Handwashing, instead of using an alcohol-based rub, is required when:
- You first arrive at the facility
- Hands are visibly dirty
- Hands have been in contact with bodily fluids or have touched items that may have been contaminated with bodily fluids
- Caring for patients with certain infections
- Before you go on break and before you leave your shift
- Before and after eating, drinking, smoking, putting on contact lenses
- Aftering using the restroom, coughing, sneezing, blowing your nose, touching your hair, or applying makeup

Skill: Hand Washing
1. Wet hands and wrists with warm water and then apply soap.
2. **Lather all surfaces of wrists, hands, and fingers producing friction, for at least 30 seconds, keeping hands lower than the elbow. Keep fingertips down and lower than the wrist.**
3. Clean fingernails by rubbing fingertips against the palms of the opposite hand.
4. **Rinse all surfaces of wrists, hands, and fingers, keeping hands lower than the elbows and fingertips down.**
5. Use clean paper towel to dry wrist, hands, and fingers, starting at the fingertips.
6. Throw paper towel into trash can.
7. Use a clean paper towel to turn off the faucet.
8. Do not touch the inside of the sink at any time.

Gloves

- Wear gloves when there is the possibility of being in contact with blood, body fluids, mucous membranes, broken skin, etc.
- Change gloves when moving from a contaminated body part to a clean body part.

- Remove gloves when you're done with a patient and wash your hands.
- Gloves should be removed before recording a procedure.

Personal Protective Equipment (PPE)

- Wear a mask, eye protection, face shields, and gowns if there is a risk of being splashed with blood or other bodily fluids.
- Wear personal protective equipment if an infectious disease is suspected, even if the diagnosis has not been confirmed yet.

Skill: Putting On PPE

1. Remove watch and all jewelry.
2. Wash and dry hands.
3. Put on a gown with the opening at the back; tie the neck and waist strings. Make sure the gown is snug and covers your uniform.
4. Put on a mask or respirator. Place the mask so that it covers your nose and mouth; tie the mask at the back of your head.
5. Put on goggles or a face shield.
6. Put on gloves. Make sure that the glove cuffs cover the gown cuffs.

Skill: Removing PPE

1. **Before removing gown, remove gloves. Remove the first glove by grabbing the glove from the outside and turning it inside out. Use two ungloved fingers to reach inside the other glove and turn it inside out. Throw away the gloves.**
2. Wash hands.
3. Remove goggles or face shield. Lift the headbands to remove the goggles or face shield; do not touch the front of goggles or face shield. The front of goggles/masks are considered contaminated.
4. Remove the gown. Do not touch the outside of the gown.
   a. Untie neck and waist strings.
   b. Without touching the outside of the gown, pull the gown inside out, down, and hold the gown away from you. Do not let the gown touch the floor.
   c. Keep gown inside out and throw it away in a biohazardous waste container; do not put it on the floor.
5. Remove the mask. Untie the strings and remove the mask by grasping only the ties. Throw away the mask.
6. If a respirator was worn, remove the respirator after leaving the room.
7. Wash hands.

Sharp Objects

- Keep needles and sharp objects away from patients when not in use.
- Do not force needles, syringes, and sharp objects into containers.
- Never empty sharp containers.

- Be careful when changing linens because there may be discarded needles.
- Promptly report any accidental needle stick or puncture wound.

Equipment

- Shared equipment should be cleaned and sterilized. To clean equipment:
    - Wear PPE if cleaning equipment that is contaminated with bodily fluids.
    - Work from clean to dirty areas. Scrub with soap and hot water.
    - Rinse items in cold water; hot water makes organic matter sticky and hard to remove.
    - Disinfect the equipment or send it to be sterilized. Disinfect the sink.
- To disinfect equipment or the sink:
    - Use a disinfectant (a chemical that kills many pathogens)
- To sterilize (kill all pathogens) items, use one of the following methods:
    - Boiled water, radiation, chemicals, autoclave (pressure steam sterilizer).

Environment

- Keep areas clutter free to prevent patients from tripping over items.
- Wipe and disinfect spills immediately.
- Follow established procedures for cleaning, removing, and disposing hazardous waste. Hazardous waste must be discarded in a designated biohazard container.

Linens

- Always hold linen away from the your body; your clothing is considered dirty.
- Do not shake linens because that can spread microbes.
- Do not let linen touch the floor; linens that touch the floor need to be changed promptly.
- Soiled linen should be removed immediately. To remove soiled linen:
    - Fold contaminated side inward; put the soiled linen inside a plastic bag, tie the bag, and put the bag in the soiled linen area.

Contact Precautions

- Used for patients with known or suspected infections that are transmitted through contact.
- Keep patient in a single room if possible. If not possible; keep privacy curtain between beds closed.
- Limit transporting patient out of the room unless necessary.

Droplet Precautions

- Used for patients with known or suspected infections that are transmitted through respiratory droplets.
- Keep patient in a single room if possible. If not possible; keep privacy curtain between beds closed.

- Limit transporting patient out of the room unless necessary.
- Wear a mask when entering the patient's room.

Airborne Precautions

- Used for patients with known or suspected infections that are transmitted by airborne particles (tuberculosis, smallpox, SARS, etc.)
- Keep patient in an airborne infection isolation room. If one is not available, the patient should be transferred to a facility that has an isolation room.
- Everyone entering the isolation room must wear a respirator.
- Doors must be closed at all times and treatments are done inside the isolation room.
- If the patient must be transferred out of the room, the patient must wear a surgical mask. Staff transporting the patient do not need to wear a mask or respirator.

Bloodborne Pathogen Standards

- Bloodborne pathogens are transmitted through blood and other potentially infectious materials (OPIM) such as semen, vaginal secretions, cerebrospinal fluids, wound drainages, and other body fluids. Unless visible blood is present, the following body fluids are NOT considered to be potentially infectious: feces, nasal secretions, saliva, sputum, sweat, tears, urine, vomitus.
- Staff members should receive training on how to reduce exposure to bloodborne pathogens and what to do if they are exposed.
- Staff members should receive all necessary vaccinations.

Surgery

- Do not touch equipment or other items that are in the sterile field (area free of all pathogens); if items in a sterile field are touched, it is considered contaminated.

Interpersonal Skills

- Greet patient and introduce yourself. Address the patient by name.
- Provide explanations before beginning and throughout a procedure.
- Protect the patients privacy by closing doors and protect the patient's body from undue exposure.

Lifting and Moving Patients

To safely lift and move patients, do the following:

- Always check the care plan for any precautions you need to take before moving a patient.
- Always explain to the patient what you are going to do before doing it.
- Reduce the height or distance a patient needs to be moved.
- Face the patient and keep the patient as close to the body as possible.
- Use both arms, your legs, hip, gluteal, and abdominal muscles. Do not use your back muscles. Avoid twisting at the waist.
- When moving the patient's body, move the top first, than torso, and then the legs. In certain situations, you may need to log roll (roll the patient as a single unit, keeping the neck and spine as straight and still as possible) the patient.
- Ask for assistance and/or use mechanical lift devices or lift sheets as needed. Mechanical lifts are used either when a patient is too heavy or unable to help with transfers.
  - Stand assist lifts are used when a patient is can bear some weight, sit up at the side of the bed with or without assistance, and bend the hips, knees, and ankles.
  - Full-sling mechanical lifts are used when patients are unable to bear weight, too heavy, or have physical limitations that prevent them from helping with transfers.
- Protect the patient's skin; friction and shearing can injure the skin and cause infections and pressure ulcers. To reduce friction and shearing when moving a patient:
  - Roll the patient
  - Use friction reducing devices such as lift/turning sheets, drawsheets, turning pads, etc.

Logrolling a Patient

Logrolling means to turn a person as a unit; keeping the head, neck, and spine aligned. It is typically used to turn patients with hip fractures, arthritic spines, and spinal injury. Two to three staff members are needed to logroll a patient.

1. Adjust the bed to a comfortable working height, make the bed as flat as possible, and lock the wheels.
2. There should be at least one CNA standing on each side of the bed.
3. Lower the rails.
4. Roll the lift sheet toward the patient's body. In unison, lift the patient to the opposite side of which the patient will be turned.
5. Place a pillow between the knees and cross the patient's arms across the chest.
6. Raise the rails and both CNAs should move to the side the patient will be turned. One person standing next to the shoulders and chest and the other person near the hips and thighs.
7. Roll the lift sheet toward the patient's body and tell the patient to keep their body rigid.

8. Grasp the lift sheet and in unison, roll the patient's body toward you.
9. Use pillows as directed by care plan and nurses to make patient comfortable.

Moving Patients Up in Bed

If a patient slides too far down in bed, it may be uncomfortable or interfere with their breathing.
1. Adjust the bed to a comfortable working height and lock the wheels. Lower the head of the bed and keep the bed as flat as possible.
2. Stand on one side of the bed while another staff members stands on the opposite side.
3. Lower the rails.
4. Remove the pillows.
5. Position a lift sheet so that it's under the patient's hip and shoulders.
6. Roll the lift sheet as close as possible towards the patient's body.
7. Both staff members should grasp the lift sheet (palms down) at the person's shoulders and hips.
8. On the count of 3 and in unison, lift (do not drag) the patient towards the head of the bed.
9. Reposition the pillows, straighten the linens, and raise the head of the bed to what the patient desires.
10. Lower the bed to its lowest position and lock the wheels.

Skill: Position Patients on Their Side

1. Perform hand hygiene and put on gloves.
2. Lower the head of the bed and raise side rail on side to which body will be turned.
3. Help the patient roll onto their side toward the raised side rail.
4. Place or adjust the pillows under the head.
5. Move the patient's arm and shoulder so that the patient is not lying on their arm.
6. Place a supportive device behind the client's back, on the top arm, and between the legs, with the top knee flexed. Support the knee and ankle.
7. Lower the bed.
8. Remove gloves and wash hands.

Moving Patients to the Side of the Bed

Moving patients to the side of the bed is typically a necessary first step in many transfer procedures.
1. Adjust the bed to comfortable working height and lock the wheels.
2. Raise the rails on the opposite side of you and then lower the rails on your side.
3. Have the patient cross their arms around the chest.
4. Move the patient's head and shoulders toward you, lifting from under the patient's neck and shoulders.
5. Move the patient's torso toward you, lifting from under the patient's waist and thighs.
6. Move the patient's lower extremities towards you, lifting from under the patient's legs.
7. Check if the patient is comfortable and raise the side rails.

Help Patients Sit on the Side of the Bed

1. Lower the side rails on your side; raise the opposite side rail.
2. Turn the patient so they are lying on their side and facing you.
3. Raise the head of the bed to a sitting position.
4. Standing by the patient's hips, place one arm under the shoulders and the other arm over the patient's thighs, near the knees.
5. Move the patient's legs over the side of the bed, while raising the patient's torso into a sitting position.
6. Support the patient in a sitting position.
7. Check if the patient feels dizzy. Check the patient's pulse and breathing.
8. Let the patient sit for as long as specified in the care plan.
9. Return the patient to bed by reversing the procedure.

Skill: Transferring a Patient from the Bed to a Chair or Wheelchair Using a Transfer Belt

1. Move the chair or wheelchair next to the patient's bed, on the patient's strong side. The wheelchair should be at the head of the bed and facing the foot or at the foot of the bed and facing the head.
2. **Raise the wheelchair footplates and lock the wheels.**
3. Lower the bed and lock the wheels.
4. Lower the side rail on your side.
5. Help the patient put on a robe and shoes.
6. **Help the patient sit on the side of the bed with their feet flat on the floor.**
7. If using a transfer belt:
    a. Wrap transfer belt around the patient's waist, over clothing.
    b. Instruct the patient to begin standing when you count to three.
    c. Stand in front of the patient, facing the patient.
    d. On the count of three, grab the transfer belt on each side in an upward motion. Stand knee to knee or toe to toe with the patient to maintain stability.
8. If not using a transfer belt:
    a. Place your hands under the patient's arms and around the patient's shoulder blades.
    b. Tell the patient to hold on to the mattress, put feet on the floor, and lean forward.
    c. Put your feet and knees against the patient's feet and knees.
    d. Tell the patient, on the count of 3, to push against the mattress as you lift them to a standing position.
9. Support the patient and help them pivot until the back of the patient's knees touch the chair or wheelchair.
10. Have the patient grasp the arms of the chair and on the count of 3, lower the patient on to the chair.
11. Position their feet on the footrests.

12. Wash hands.

Transferring a Patient Using a Stand-Assist Mechanical Lift

1. Move the chair or wheelchair next to the patient's bed, on the patient's strong side.
2. Raise the wheelchair footplates and lock the wheels.
3. Lower the bed and lock the wheels.
4. Lower the side rail on your side.
5. Help the patient put on a robe and shoes.
6. Help the patient sit on the side of the bed.
7. Apply the sling.
8. Position the lift in front of the person, widen the base for stability, and lock the wheels.
9. Have the patient place their feet on the foot plates and knees against the knee pad. Wrap strap around the knees.
10. Attach the sling to the lift.
11. Have the patient hold the lift's hand grips.
12. Unlock the lift's wheels. Use the lift to raise the patient.
13. Move the lift to the chair or wheelchair and lower the patient.
14. Lock the lift wheels.
15. Unhook the sling and remove the sling.

Transferring a Patient Using a Full-Sling Mechanical Lift

You will need two staff members to perform this procedure. Full sling mechanical lifts are used to transfer patients that are too heavy or cannot walk nor assist in the transfer.

1. Move the chair or wheelchair next to the bed.
2. Lower and flatten the bed and lock the wheels.
3. Place the lift sling under the patient.
4. Position the lift over the person.
5. Widen the lift's base for stability and lock the wheels.
6. Attach the sling to the lift.
7. Unlock the lift wheels.
8. Use the lift to raise the patient off the bed. As you are raising the patient, have another staff member guide the patient with their hands and support the patient's legs.
9. Lower the patient onto a chair or wheelchair.
10. Lock the lift wheels. Unhook the sling and remove the sling.

Transferring a Patient from a Bed to a Stretcher

At least 2 or 3 staff members to perform this procedure. If the patient is under 200 pounds, a friction reducing device (lift sheet, turning pad, drawsheet, slide sheet, lateral transfer device) is used. If the patient is over 200 pounds, 3 staff members are needed and a mechanical device is used.

1. Lower and flatten the bed and lock the wheels.
2. Lower the rails.
3. Hold onto the pull sheet at the patient's shoulder and waist while another staff member holds onto the pull sheet at the patient's hips and thighs. In unison, pull the patient towards you.
4. Move the stretcher to the side of the bed you're on. Adjust the stretcher so that it is at the same height as the bed and lock the wheels.
5. Roll the pullsheet towards the patient on both sides.
6. In unison, use the pullsheet to lift the patient onto the stretcher.
7. Secure the patient and raise the side rails of the stretcher.
8. Unlock the wheels on the stretcher and transport the patient.

Skill: Assisting With Ambulation Using A Transfer Belt

Gait or transfer belts are used to help patients who are weak, but able to walk, to stand or walk.

1. Adjust the bed to a safe and comfortable working position. Lock the wheels.
2. **Before helping a patient stand, ensure that the patient is wearing non-skid shoes/footwear and is in a sitting position with their feet flat on the ground.**
3. While the patient is still sitting, wrap the transfer belt snugly around the patient's waist, over clothing. The buckle should be in front and slightly to the side. You should be able to slide an open flat hand under the belt.
4. Tell the patient to begin standing at the count of three.
5. You should stand, facing the client.
6. Count to three to get the client to start standing. On the count of three, help the patient stand by grabbing the transfer belt on both sides and holding the belt from underneath with two hands. Stand knee to knee or toe to toe with the patient to maintain stability.
7. When walking, walk to the side and slightly behind the patient.

Taking Vital Signs

Measuring a patient's height, weight, and vital signs provides important clues to a patient's health. Vital signs include pulse, respiration, blood pressure, and temperature. Vital signs can be affected by the time of day, a patient's emotions, food intake, and many other factors. Significant changes in weight can indicate a nutritional deficiency or other disease. Loss of height can indicate musculoskeletal problems. All vital sign equipments should be cleaned after each use.

Since vital signs can be affected by stress, fear, etc., measure vital signs for young children in the following order:
1. Respirations
2. Pulse
3. Blood pressure
4. Temperature

If a child was crying, make a note of that along with the vital sign measurements.

Normal respiration and heart rates:

Population	Age	Respiration Rate	Heart Rate	Blood Pressure
Neonate	0 to 1 month	30 to 60 breaths per minute	120 to 160 beats per minute	Systolic pressure around 70
Infant	Up to 1 years old	25 to 50 breaths per minute	100 to 140 beats per minute	Systolic pressure around 90
Toddlers	1 to 2 years old	20 to 30 breaths per minute	90 to 140 beats per minute	Systolic pressure between 80 and 90
Preschoolers	3 to 5 years old	20 to 25 breaths per minute	80 to 130 beats per minute	Systolic pressure between 90 to 110
Children	6 to 11 years old	15 to 20 breaths per minute	70 to 110 beats per minute	Systolic pressure between 90 and 120
Adolescents	12 to 18 years	12 to 20 breaths	60 to 100 beats	Systolic

	old	per minute	per minute	pressure between 100 to 120
Early Adulthood	19 to 40 years old	12 to 20 breaths per minute	60 to 100 beats per minute	110/70 to 130/90
Middle Adulthood	41 to 60 years old	12 to 20 breaths per minute	60 to 100 beats per minute	110/70 to 130/90
Late Adulthood	61+ years old	Depends on health	Depends on health	Depends on health

Temperatures

The body produces heat as a normal part of metabolism (converting food into energy). Our body temperatures can vary based on physical or emotional stress, extreme heat or cold environments, activity levels, infections, etc. Thermometers are used to measure the body temperature. The following types of thermometers are used: glass thermometer, electronic thermometer, tympanic thermometer, and temporal artery thermometer. Glass thermometers are rarely used. Electronic thermometers are the most frequently used thermometers.

Febrile means a person with a fever. Afebrile means a person without a fever.

Oral Temperatures
Oral temperatures should not be taken if:
- The patient is under 4 or 5 years of age.
- The patient is unconscious.
- The patient has a sore mouth.
- The patient is receiving oxygen or breathing through the mouth.
- The patient has a seizure disorder.

When measuring oral temperature using an electric thermometer:

1. Ask the patient if they've have eaten or smoked anything within the last 15 minutes. Wait at least 15 minutes before taking oral temperatures if a patient recently smoked or drank a hot or cold liquid.
2. Remove thermometer pack from charger and attach oral probe to thermometer. Cover the oral probe with a disposable plastic probe cover.
3. Ask the patient to open their mouth and place the probe under the patient's tongue and to one side.
4. Ask the patient to close their mouth around the probe.
5. Remove the probe when you hear a beep.

6. Read the temperature.
7. Discard the plastic probe cover by pushing the eject button on the thermometer.
8. Clean the equipment and return the thermometer probe to the recording unit and return the thermometer to the charger.
9. Record the temperature along with the method used to obtain the temperature.

When measuring oral temperature using a glass thermometer:

1. Ask the patient if they've have eaten or smoked anything within the last 15 minutes. Wait at least 15 minutes before taking oral temperatures if a patient recently smoked or drank a hot or cold liquid.
2. Rinse the thermometer with cool water if the thermometer was sitting in a disinfectant. Dry the thermometer and check for any cracks; discard the thermometer if there are any cracks. Shake the thermometer until the substance is below 94F. Cover with a thermometer sheath.
3. Ask the patient to open their mouth and place the probe under the patient's tongue and to one side.
4. Ask the patient to close their mouth around the probe. Leave it in the mouth for 3 to 5 minutes or follow facility policies.
5. Remove the thermometer from the patient's mouth. Remove and discard the thermometer sheath. Read the temperature by holding the thermometer horizontally, at eye level.
6. Clean the thermometer and store it in a container with disinfectant solution. Do not use hot water to clean the thermometer; hot water causes the substance to expand, breaking the thermometer.
7. Record the temperature along with the method used to obtain the temperature.

Rectal Temperatures
Rectal temperatures are taken when oral temperatures cannot be taken and/or the patient is under 3 years old. Rectal temperatures should not be taken if:
- The patient has diarrhea.
- The patient has heart disease.
- The patient has a rectal disorder or injury.

When measuring rectal temperature using an electronic thermometer:
1. Perform hand hygiene and put on gloves.
2. Raise the side rails, flatten the bed as much as tolerated, and have the patient lie on their side so they are facing away from you.
3. Fan-fold the top linens to below the patient's buttocks. Expose buttocks while keeping the rest of the body covered.
4. Remove the thermometer pack from charger and attach the rectal probe to the thermometer.
5. Cover the rectal probe with a disposable plastic probe cover.

6. Apply lubricant to a tissue and cover at least 1 to 2 inches of the probe with lubricant.
7. Separate the buttocks using your non-dominant hand and tell the patient to breathe slowly and relax.
8. Use your dominant hand to insert 1 to 2 inches of the probe into the anus; aim the probe towards the umbilicus. Do not force the probe. If you feel resistance, stop and notify a nurse.
9. Remove the probe when you hear a beep.
10. Wipe the anal area to remove lubricant and feces; discard the tissue in a biohazardous receptacle.
11. Read the temperature.
12. Discard the plastic probe cover by pushing the eject button on the thermometer.
13. Remove and discard gloves. Perform hand hygiene.
14. Bring top-linens over the patient and adjust the bed so that the patient is comfortable.
15. Clean the equipment and return the thermometer probe to the recording unit and return the thermometer to the charger.
16. Record the temperature along with the method used to obtain the temperature.

When measuring rectal temperature using a glass thermometer:
1. Perform hand hygiene and put on gloves.
2. Raise the side rails, flatten the bed as much as tolerated, and have the patient lie on their side so they are facing away from you.
3. Fan-fold the top linens to below the patient's buttocks. Expose buttocks while keeping the rest of the body covered.
4. Rinse the thermometer with cool water if the thermometer was sitting in a disinfectant. Dry the thermometer and check for any cracks; discard the thermometer if there are any cracks. Shake the thermometer until the substance is below 94F. Cover with a thermometer sheath.
5. Apply lubricant to a tissue and cover at least 1 to 2 inches of the probe with lubricant.
6. Separate the buttocks using your non-dominant hand and tell the patient to breathe slowly and relax.
7. Use your dominant hand to insert 1 to 2 inches of the probe into the anus; aim the probe towards the umbilicus. Do not force the probe. If you feel resistance, stop and notify a nurse.
8. Leave the thermometer in for 3 to 5 minutes or follow facility policies.
9. Remove the thermometer and wipe the anal area to remove lubricant and feces; discard the tissue in a biohazardous receptacle.
10. Remove and discard the thermometer sheath. Read the temperature by holding the thermometer horizontally, at eye level.
11. Discard the plastic probe cover by pushing the eject button on the thermometer.
12. Remove and discard gloves. Perform hand hygiene.
13. Bring top-linens over the patient and adjust the bed so that the patient is comfortable.

14. Clean the thermometer and store it in a container with disinfectant solution. Do not use hot water to clean the thermometer; hot water causes the substance to expand, breaking the thermometer.
15. Record the temperature along with the method used to obtain the temperature.

Axillary Temperatures

Axillary (underarm) temperature is the least accurate temperature; only take axillary temperature if other sites cannot be used.

When measuring axillary temperature using an electric thermometer:

Make sure the underarms are dry and record the reading with an 'A' for axillary.
1. Remove thermometer pack from charger and attach probe to thermometer.
2. Cover probe with disposable plastic probe cover.
3. Have the patient raise their arm.
4. Hold the thermometer horizontal to the underarms and place the thermometer in the center of the underarms. Lower the patient's arm and place the arm across the patient's chest.
5. Remove the probe when you hear a beep.
6. Discard the plastic probe cover by pushing the eject button on the thermometer.
7. Clean the equipment and return the thermometer probe to the recording unit and return the thermometer to the charger.
8. Record the temperature along with the method used to obtain the temperature.

When measuring axillary temperature using a glass thermometer:
Make sure the underarms are dry and record the reading with an 'A' for axillary.
1. Rinse the thermometer with cool water if the thermometer was sitting in a disinfectant. Dry the thermometer and check for any cracks; discard the thermometer if there are any cracks. Shake the thermometer until the substance is below 94F. Cover with a thermometer sheath.
2. Have the patient raise their arm.
3. Hold the thermometer horizontal to the underarms and place the thermometer in the center of the underarms. Lower the patient's arm and place the arm across the patient's chest.
4. Leave the thermometer in for 10 minutes or follow facility policies.
5. Remove the thermometer from the patient's underarm. Remove and discard the thermometer sheath. Read the temperature by holding the thermometer horizontally, at eye level.
6. Clean the thermometer and store it in a container with disinfectant solution. Do not use hot water to clean the thermometer; hot water causes the substance to expand, breaking the thermometer.
7. Record the temperature along with the method used to obtain the temperature.

Tympanic Temperatures

Tympanic temperature should not be taken if the patient has an ear disorder or ear drainage. If the patient wears a hearing aid, remove the hearing aid and wait at least 2 minutes before taking their temperature.

When measuring tympanic (ear) temperature:
1. Have the patient turn their head to one side.
2. Note if there is visible earwax in the ear canal opening and wipe away excess earwax; do not remove earwax from anything inside the outer ear canal.
3. Remove thermometer from the charger.
4. Cover the speculum with a disposable cover.
5. Gently pull the top of the ear up and back (for adults) or straight back (for children) and then insert speculum.
6. Remove the probe when you hear a beep.
7. Discard the plastic speculum cover by pushing the eject button on the thermometer.
8. Clean the equipment and return the thermometer probe to the recording unit and return the thermometer to the charger.
9. Record the temperature along with the method used to obtain the temperature.

Temporal Artery (Forehead) Temperatures

When measuring forehead temperature:
1. Remove hair and any other coverings away from the forehead.
2. Cover the probe with a disposable cover.
3. Hold the "ON" button and place the probe on the center of the forehead. Still holding the "ON" button, slide the probe, horizontally, across the forehead to the hairline.
4. With the "ON" button still pressed, place the probe on the neck, behind the ear lobe.
5. Release the "ON" button and read the temperature.
6. Remove and discard the cover.
7. Record the temperature along with the method used to obtain the temperature.

Blood Pressure

Blood pressure is the amount of pressure placed against arterial walls by blood. The systolic blood pressure tells you the pressure in your arteries when your heart contracts. Diastolic pressure tells you the pressure when your heart is at rest, between beats.

Skill: Measure and Record Manual Blood Pressure
1. Let the patient rest for 5 minutes before taking their blood pressure. Tell them to not talk because talking can raise the blood pressure.

2. Have the patient sit or lie down. If sitting, patients should have both feet flat on the ground. The patient's arms should be at the heart level or below if sitting; if lying down, the patient's arms should be at their side. Palms should be up.
3. Check that the manometer reads "0" when there is no air in the cuff.
4. Choose the proper cuff size; a cuff that is too small will result in a higher reading, a cuff that is too large will result in a lower reading.
5. Place the cuff, two finger widths above the elbow, around the patient's bare arms; clothing can affect blood pressure readings because they distort the Korotkoff sounds (blood flow sounds).
6. Place the stethoscope diaphragm over the brachial artery (in the bend of the elbow). Do not place it under the cuff.
7. Close the cuff pump valve and inflate the cuff until you can't hear the pulse. This is the systolic pressure.
8. Continue to inflate the cuff 30 mmHg more and then slowly release the pressure valve at a rate of 2 to 3 mmHg/second.
9. When you hear the first pulse sound, note the reading on the manometer; this is the systolic pressure. Continue listening until the you hear nothing; note the reading on the manometer, this is the diastolic pressure.
10. Wash hands.
11. Record blood pressure.

Notes:
- For new patients, initial blood pressure reading should be taken in both arms; record each measurement. Subsequent blood pressure measurement should be taken in the arm with the highest reading.
- Do not take blood pressure in an arm
    - That is on the same side as a masectomy
    - That has been affected by a stroke or is injured or malformed
    - That has a current IV or shunt in it

Pulse

Arteries carry blood away from the heart and to the body. Veins return blood to the heart. Pulse rate is the number of heartbeats in 1 minute. Tachycardia is a heart rate of more than 100 beats per minutes. Bradycardia is a heart rate of less than 60 beats per minute. The pulse rate can be taken from the following pulse sites:
- carotid pulse: pulse on carotid artery in neck
- femoral pulse: pulse on femoral artery in groin
- radial pulse: pulse on wrist
- apical pulse: pulse on the tip of the heart
- brachial pulse: pulse near upper arm beneath biceps or inside of elbow
- dorsalis pedis: pulse on top of foot

Skill: Taking the Radial (Wrist) Pulse
1. Have the patient sit or lie down.
2. If the patient is lying down, place their arm straight at their side or fold their arm over the chest. If the patient is sitting down, have them place their arm on a flat surface or support their arm with your arms.
3. Place your first two fingers on the thumb side of the patient's wrist.
4. Note if the pulse is strong or weak and regular or irregular.
5. Count the pulse for 30 seconds and multiply by 2. If the patient has heart disease or the pulse rate is irregular or less than 60 beats per minute, count the pulse for 60 seconds..
6. If the pulse rate is less than 60 BPM or greater than 100 BPM, notify the nurse.
7. Wash hands.
8. Record the rate, strength, type of pulse taken, and regularity of the pulse rate.

When measuring the apical (at apex of the heart) pulse:
1. Clean stethoscope earpieces and diaphragm.
2. Have patient lie down or sit.
3. Expose the left side of the chest and sternum.
4. Use your fingers to locate the apical pulse. Place the stethoscope over the apical pulse.
5. Count pulse for 60 seconds.
6. If the pulse rate is less than 60 BPM or greater than 100 BPM, notify the nurse.
7. Cover up the patient.
8. Clean the stethoscope earpieces and diaphragm.
9. Record the rate, strength, type of pulse taken, and regularity of the pulse rate.

Respiration

Respiration involves inhalation and exhalation. During inhalation, the chest expands (rises) as air is breathed in. During exhalation, the chest falls as air is breathed out. When measuring respiration, pay attention to the rate, rhythm, depth (shallow or deep breaths), and ease of respiration (wheezing, rattling, etc.). Changes in respiration can indicate a disease or life-threatening condition.

Skill: Counting Respirations
1. Have the patient sit or lie down.
2. Place your hand on the patient's chest or upper abdomen.
3. Count breaths for 1 minute. One inhale plus one exhale equals one breath.
4. Wash hands.
5. Record the rate, depth, and ease of breathing.

Pulse Oximetry

Pulse oximetry measures the oxygen concentration in the blood. A reading of 95 to 100% is normal. When measuring pulse oximetry in adults, attach the sensor to the adult's finger. When measuring pulse oximetry in young children, attach the sensor to the sole of the foot, palm of the hand, or toe. If the patient, young or old, moves a lot or has tremors, shivers, or seizures, attach the sensor to the earlobe.

Bright lights, nail polish, fake nails, and movements may affect measurements.
- Place a towel over the sensor to block bright lights.
- Remove nail polish or fake nails; otherwise, use a different site.
- Do not measure blood pressure on the side the pulse oximetry sensor is attached to because blood pressure cuffs affect blood flow.

Measuring Height and Weight

A patient's weight and height are measured upon admission to a facility and on a routine basis. Changes in weight and height can provide clues into a person's overall health. Try to weigh patients at the same time of day, wearing the same type of clothing with no shoes, and after they've emptied their bladder.

Measuring Height and Weight Using an Upright Scale

Skill: Measure and Record Weight of Ambulatory Patient

An upright scale is used to measure the weight and height of patients that can stand. It has a lower and upper bar; the lower bar is divided into 50 lbs and the upper bar is divided into fractions of a pound. Add the upper and lower bar values to determine a patient's weight. For example, is the lower bar weight is at 100 lbs and the upper bar weight is at 10 lbs; the patient's weight is 100 + 10 = 110 lbs.

1. Ensure the patient has non-skid shoes/footwear on.
2. Ask the patient to empty their bladder.
3. Move the lower and upper weights to 0.
4. Ask the patient to stand on the scale; do not allow them to hold on to you or anything else.
5. Move the upper and lower weights until the balance pointer is in the middle. Note the patient's weight.
6. Lower or extend the height rod so that it's on top of the patient's head. Note the patient's height.
7. Wash hands.
8. Record weight and height.

Measuring Height and Weight Using a Chair Scale

A chair scale is used to measure the height and weight of a patients that can't stand, but can get out of bed; they are also used for patients in wheelchairs.

1. Ask the patient to empty their bladder.
2. Set scale to 0.
3. Help the patient onto the scale.
   a. If a regular chair scale is being used, transfer the patient onto the chair. The patient's buttocks should be against the back of the chair and their feet on the footrests.
   b. If using a wheelchair scale, push the patient and wheelchair onto the scale and lock the wheelchair.

4. Note the weight. If using a wheelchair, subtract the weight of the empty wheelchair from the total weight.

Measuring Height and Weight in Bed

A sling scale is used to measure the weight of patients that can't get out of bed. A tape measure is used to measure the height of patients that can't get out of bed.

1. Ask the patient to empty their bladder.
2. Position the sling scale next to the bed. Lock the wheels of the bed and lower the rail on the side you are working on.
3. Fanfold top linens to the foot of the bed.
4. Place the sling under the patient.
5. Close the release valve on the sling scale.
6. Raise the sling scale so that it is over the patient.
7. To provide stability, spread the legs of the sling scale and lock the legs. If you don't lock the legs, the scale could tip over.
8. Hook the sling to the scale; make sure hooks are faced away from the person.
9. Slowly raise the sling and read the weight on the screen.
10. Lower the scale and remove the sling from under the patient.
11. To measure the patient's height (patient is in supine position):
    a. Have a coworker hold the beginning of the tape measure at the patient's heel.
    b. Pull the other end of the tape measure until it extends a few inches past the head.
    c. Place a ruler flat against the patient's head and over the tape measure.
    d. Note where the lower edge of the ruler touches the tape measure; this is the patient's height.

Bedmaking

Closed bed: a bed that is not in use; top linens are not folded back.

Open bed: a bed that is in use; top linens are folded back.

Occupied bed: a bed with a person in it.

Surgical bed: bed made to transfer a person from a stretcher to a bed.

Making a Closed Bed

1. Put on gloves.
2. Collect supplies and place them on a clean surface.
3. Adjust the bed height to what is comfortable for you to work with. Ensure the bed as flat as possible and wheels are locked.
4. Remove linens by rolling each sheet away from you. Put disposable sheets in the trash and dirty linens in designated hampers.
5. Clean the bed and frame if that is part of your duties.
6. Place mattress pad on the bed.
7. Place bottom sheet on top of the mattress pad; unfold lengthwise and ensure the center crease is in the middle of the bed. Miter the corners.
8. Tuck sheet under the mattress, starting from the head to the foot of the bed.
9. Place a cotton or waterproof draw sheet on the bed; unfold lengthwise and ensure the center crease is in the middle of the bed. Tuck sheet under the mattress.
10. Go to the other side of the bed.
11. Tuck bottom sheet and draw sheet under the mattress; mitre the corners.
12. Place top sheet on the bed and unfold lengthwise, ensure the center crease is in the middle of the bed. Follow the same steps to apply the blanket and then the bedspread.
13. Tuck the topsheet, blanket, and bedspread together at the foot of the bed. Miter the corner and leave sides untucked. Go to the otherside of the bed and repeat the steps.
14. Turn back the top sheet over the blanket and spread to form a cuff.
15. Put pillowcases on pillows and place pillows on the bed.

Making an Open Bed

1. Follow the same procedures for making a closed bed; except top linens are folded back.

Making an Occupied Bed

1. Check the care plan to see if any precautions need to be taken when moving the patient.
2. Put on gloves.
3. Collect supplies and place them on a clean surface.
4. Adjust the bed height to what is comfortable for you to work with. Ensure the bed is as flat as possible and wheels are locked..
5. Lower the side rail, only on the side you are working on.

6. Loosen the top bed linens at the foot of the bed.
7. Fold and remove the bedspread; then do the same for the blanket. Place the bedspread and blanket over a chair for later reuse.
8. Cover the patient with a bath blanket, for warmth and privacy, before removing the top sheet; have the patient hold the top of the bath blanket or tuck it under the patient's shoulders. Bring the top sheet, under the bath blanket, down to the patient's ankles and place it in the linen hamper.
9. Have the patient turn, or turn the patient, on their side so they are facing away from you.
10. Loosen bottom linens, beneath the patient, from the top of the bed to the foot of the bed. Fan fold the bottom linens, including the mattress pad and starting with the drawsheet, toward the patient and tuck them under the patient. If reusing the mattress pad, do not fan fold it.
11. Disinfect and dry the exposed mattress surface if soiled.
12. If using a new mattress pad, place it on the bed and unfold it lengthwise. Ensure that the center crease is in the middle. Fanfold the top of the mattress pad toward the patient.
13. Clean and dry the exposed mattress, if soiled.
14. Apply clean linen to the exposed side of the bed, mattress pad first, placing the center creases lengthwise along the center of the bed and fanfold other half toward the patient; do the same thing with the bottom sheet, then pull sheet.
15. Roll the patient towards you, explaining to them that they will roll over the linens on the bed and feel a bump.
16. Raise the side rail and move to the opposite side and lower the rails.
17. Loosen bottom linens and remove them one at a time. Place disposable products in the trash; place dirty linens in designated hampers.
18. Change gloves if soiled.
19. Pull clean bottom sheets toward you and tuck sheets under the bed from the head to the foot of the bed. Do the same with the pull sheet.
20. Position the patient, on their back, in the center of the bed.
21. Place top sheet, over the patient and bath blanket, and unfold lengthwise; ensure that the center crease is in the middle of the bed.
22. Have the patient hold the top sheet or tuck it under their shoulders and remove the bath blanket from under the top sheet.
23. Place a blanket on the bed and unfold lengthwise; ensure the center crease is in the middle of the bed. The top of the blanket should be 6 to 8 inches below the top of the mattress.
24. Place a bedspread on the bed and unfold lengthwise; ensure the center crease is in the middle of the bed and the top of the bedspread is aligned with the top of the mattress.
25. Turn back the top sheet over the blanket and spread to form a cuff.
26. Go to the foot of the bed and make a toe pleat to relieve pressure and allow the patient to move their to feet. To make a toe pleat, hold the bedspread, blanket, and top sheet together and pull straight up about 2 inches.
27. Tuck all top linens under the bottom of the mattress, leaving the sides untucked.
28. Raise the rail.

29. Change the pillowcases.

Make a Surgical Bed

1. Practice hand hygiene and put on gloves.
2. Remove all linens from the bed and place them in the laundry hamper.
3. Remove gloves, practice hand hygiene, and put on new gloves.
4. Make a closed bed, except do not tuck the top linens under the bed.
5. Fold top linens at the foot of the bed back onto the bed.
6. Fan fold linens lengthwise to the side opposite the side the stretcher will be on.
7. Leave the bed in the highest position and leave both bed rails down.

Safety

Falls

Falls are one of the most common accidents. Always be on alert for scenarios that can cause a patient to fall. To help prevent falls:
- Clean up and dry wet floors immediately. Place signs when floors are wet.
- Remove equipment or items that are in walking paths.
- Do not use throw rugs; floors should be 1 solid color as prints can cause dizziness in elders.
- Use equipment properly and do not use damaged equipment.
- Provide adequate lighting.
- Make sure patients wear glasses, use canes, etc. if necessary.
- Keep call lights and frequently used supplies within easy reach of patients.
- Keep patient beds in the lowest position
- Use safety bars in showers, tubs, and near toilets.

If a patient complains of dizziness, help them sit in a chair; if a chair is not close by, help them sit on the floor. If a patient is falling, do not try to prevent the fall; you may injure yourself and the patient. Instead, place your body behind the person and wrap your arounds around the torso; ease the patient to the floor by letting them slide down your body, while protecting their head. Before moving the person, wait for the nurse to assess if the patient is injured.

Identification

It is extremely important you correctly identify and treat the correct patient. Always check a patient's wristband before serving meals or medication or performing any type of care on them. Use at least 2 identifiers.

Hazardous Chemicals

Hazardous chemicals are chemicals that can cause a health or physical hazard. They are required to having warning labels on the container; the warning label contains the manufacturer info, product identifier, hazard severity ("Danger", "Warning"), and hazard statements ("Harmful if swallowed", etc.). Do not use a substance if the warning label is removed or damaged.

All hazardous chemicals are required to have a Safety Data Sheet (SDS). Safety Data Sheet contains information about the chemical, including what to do if someone is exposed to the chemical or there is a leak. Check the SDS before using a chemical, cleaning up a spill, or disposing the substance. Never leave a leak or spill unattended.

Preventing Poisoning
- Keep harmful products locked up in hard to reach areas.

- Use prescriptions drugs correctly.
- Buy products with child resistant packaging.
- Do not store harmful products near food.

Preventing Burns

- Keep patients away from stoves, grills, fireplaces, furnaces, etc.
- Keep hot food and liquids away from counter and table edges.
- Do not pour hot liquids near patients.
- Assist with eating and drinking as needed.
- Do not allow the use of space heaters.
- Do not let patients sleep with a heating pad or electric blanket.
- Do not leaving smoking materials at the bedside.
- No smoking near oxygen tanks.

Fire

Remember the R.A.C.E acronym for fire evacuations.
- Remove all residents in the immediate area of a fire.
- Activate the fire alarm.
- Contain the fire by closing all doors and windows in the area of a fire. Turn off oxygen and electrical items near the fire.
- Extinguish the fire (if the fire is small enough).

Abuse

Be on the lookout for signs of abuse or neglect and report any concerns you have to your supervisor.

Signs and symptoms of abuse in the elderly include:
- Bruises
- Bleeding beneath the scalp from hair pulling
- Cigarette burns
- Rope marks
- Lacerations
- Trauma injuries.

It is also important to recognize and report signs of physical abuse in children such as:
- Bruises and burns in unusual shapes and locations. It's common for children to trip and hurt their shins, foreheads, and chins. Injuries to the torso (back or front), upper arms or legs, and genitalia are more suspicious. Burns without splash marks are also suspicious.
- Injury doesn't match with cause provided
- Multiple injuries in various stages of healing
- More injuries than usual

Bed Safety

A patient's head, neck, chest, arms, and legs can become entrapped within the following zones and cause serious injury and/or death:

- Within the rails
- The space between the top of a mattress and the bottom of a rail
- The space between the side of a mattress and the rail
- The space between the top of a mattress and the bottom of rail, at the end of the rail
- The space between the split bed rails
- The space between the end of a rail and edge of the headboard or footboard
- The space between the mattress end and the headboard or footboard

Children can also become entrapped within cribs. To prevent entrapment, make sure that there are no gaps between:

- The crib rail and mattress
- The crib rail and headboard
- The crib rail and footboard

Safe Restraint Usage

Restraints should never to be used to punish a patient or for staff convenience; restraints should only be used as a last resort and only to protect the patient or others from harm. A doctor's order is required for the use of restraints. Restraints can be physical or chemical. Physical restraints are devices that restrict a person's movement; examples include bed rails that prevent a person from getting out of bed, chairs placed so close to a wall that a patient cannot get out, etc. Drugs that control behavior, restrict movement, or are not standard treatment for a patient's condition can be considered chemical restraints.

Vest restraints are used to prevent patients from falling out of a bed or chair. The flaps of the vest should be crossed in front of the person's chest; it should never be backwards (back of vest on person's chest and flaps crossed a patient's back). A backwards vest can strangle a patient if the patient slides down.

Wrist restraints or mitt restraints are used to prevent a patient from removing tubes or catheters. Mitt restraints restrict finger movement while allowing more arm movement.

Lap restraints are used to prevent a person from sliding out of a chair. Waist/belt restraints are used to prevent patients from sliding out of a chair or bed.

Informed consent must be given before restraints are used. The patient must be informed of the reason for the restraints and the risks associated with it; it is the responsibility of the nurse or doctor to get the consent from the patient or legal guardian.

If a person has the physical and mental ability to release the fastener of a device, that device is NOT considered to be a restraint. For example, safety straps that a patient can unfasten if they desire are not considered restraints.

When applying restraints:
- Read and follow manufacturer instructions on how to use the restraints.
- Apply the restraints with enough help to protect the patient and staff from injury.
- Any restraint that is tied should be tied with a "quick-release knot" or "slip knot" to quickly free a person during an emergency.
- Observe the patient at least every 15 minutes or as often as directed by the nurse. Observe for signs of increased confusion or agitation. Check breathing and circulation.
- At least every 2 hours or as directed by the nurse, release the patient for at least 10 minutes, reposition the patient, and provide basic needs (fluids, food, elimination, etc.) to the patient.

Incident Reporting

An incident is any event that harmed or could harm a patient, visitor, or staff member. All incidents must be verbally reported to the nurse immediately. In addition, you must fill out an incident or accident report if you were directly involved in the incident or witnessed the incident. Incident reports are used by the facility to determine how future incidents may be prevented.

Basic Emergency Care

Immediately call emergency medical services.

CPR

Without enough oxygen, cardiac arrest and/or brain damage begins within about 4 minutes; permanent brain damage within 6 minutes; death is likely within 10 minutes. High quality chest compression and timely defibrillation are the most important factors in resuscitation.

Choking/Foreign Body Airway Obstruction (FBAO)

FBAO is when any object obstructs the airway. Signs of airway blockages include inability to cough or speak. Treat by bending the patient forward at the waist, supporting the patient's chest with one hand, while using the heel of the other hand to give 5 back blows between the shoulder blades. If that does not dislodge the object, give 5 abdominal thrusts. Abdominal thrusts, also called Heimlich Maneuver, are performed by:
1. wrapping your arms around the patient's waist,
2. placing your fist, thumb side in, just above the patient's navel
3. grab your fist with the other hand
4. make quick, inward and upward thrusts

Alternate between back blows and abdominal thrusts until object is dislodged or patient loses consciousness. If the patient loses consciousness, begin CPR starting with chest compressions. Chest compressions should be given even if the patient has a pulse, so don't waste time checking for a pulse. Before giving rescue breaths or ventilation, look inside the mouth for any visible foreign objects. If the foreign object is visible, remove it. Rescue breaths may be ineffective and not needed if the airway obstruction is complete and cannot be removed.

FBAO in Pediatric Patients

Children commonly choke on small toys as well as foods such as hot dogs, popcorn, and nuts.

In children under 1 years old:
1. Using your thigh for support, lay the infant face down, along your forearm. Ensure the patient's head is lower than the body. Use your thumb and fingers to hold the jaw.
2. Using the heel of your hand, give 5 firm back flows between the shoulder blades.
3. If the object is not dislodged after the back blows, give the baby 5 chest thrusts. Turn the baby over so that the baby is faced up. Place 2 to 3 fingers in the middle of the baby's chest, just below the nipples. Push down about 1.5 inches.
4. Alternate between back blows and chest thrusts until object is dislodged or baby loses consciousness. If the baby loses consciousness, begin CPR. Before giving rescue breaths, check for any blockages in the baby's mouth. Remove object with a straight blade laryngoscope and forcep if you can see it; if you can't see it, do not try to remove it or you may end up pushing the object further down.

In children over 1 year old, follow the same procedures as adults: alternate 5 back blows and 5 abdominal thrusts.

Mouth to Mouth/Mouth to Nose

Mouth to mouth is performed in situations where the patient does not have adequate breathing and artificial ventilation devices are not available.

- Open the airway using the head-tilt/chin thrust or jaw thrust maneuver.
- If available, put a barrier device between your mouth and the patient's mouth before giving mouth to mouth.
- In mouth to mouth, the provider forms a seal around the patient's mouth with the provider's mouth, pinches the nose, and blows air into the patient's mouth. Mouth to nose resuscitation can be used in place of mouth to mouth in cases where the patient has lower facial injuries, the patient has vomited, or the provider does not have a barrier for the mouth.
- If you do not see the chest rise and fall when giving breaths, check for FBAO.
- Give 1 breath every 5 to 6 seconds for adults; 1 breath every 3 seconds for pediatric patients.
- Mouth to mouth should be performed along with chest compressions, except in cases where chest compressions are not needed (i.e. patient's heart is beating on its own)

Chest Compressions

If a patient is in cardiac arrest, chest compressions should be performed at a rate of 100 compressions a minute. Allow full recoil between compressions. Chest compression should take precedence over rescue breaths if both cannot be done. In two provider CPR, you do not need to stop compressions to give breaths. Minimize chest compression interruptions to a maximum of 10 seconds. A good way to check if the chest compressions are deep enough is to feel for a carotid or femoral pulse with each compression. The compression to breath ratios are as follows:

Population	2 Provider Compression/Breath Ratio	1 Provider Compression/Breath Ratio	Compression Depth
Under 1 years old	15 compressions, 2 breaths	30 compressions, 2 breaths	One third anterior-posterior chest diameter (1.5 inches to 4 cm)
1 to 8 years old	15 compressions, 2 breaths	30 compressions, 2 breaths	One third anterior-posterior chest diameter (2

			inches to 5 cm)
Over 8 years old	30 compressions, 2 breaths	30 compressions, 2 breaths	2 inches

To perform a chest compression:
1. Move patient to a hard and flat surface
2. Place the heel of one hand over the center of the person's chest, between the nipples. Place your other hand on top of the first hand. Keep your elbows straight and position your shoulders directly above your hands.
3. Use your upper body weight (not just your arms) as you push straight down on the chest.

Automated External Defibrillator (AED)

An AED is a portable device that can check a heart's rhythm and deliver a shock to the heart to restore a normal rhythm. It should only be used on patients without a pulse. In addition to written instructions, AED devices also provide audio instructions when turned on.

Manual defibrillation is preferred for patients under 1 years old for better control over the amount of energy delivered. However, manual defibrillation can only be performed by Advanced Life Support (ALS); so if ALS is not on the scene, proceed with the use of a pediatric or adult AED.

If you did not witness the cardiac arrest, give 5 cycles of 30 compressions and 2 breaths before defibrillating; this will provide more oxygen to the blood so that defibrillation will be more successful. If you did witness the cardiac arrest, you should begin CPR with chest compressions while someone else prepares and applies the AED. If only one rescue provider is available, apply the AED immediately.

Below are instructions on how to use an AED:
1. Use scissors to cut patient's clothing to expose the chest. Chest should be completely bare in males and females.
2. Remove all metal objects, including jewelry and undergarments with metal components.
3. Dry chest if wet. If chest is very hairy, use a razor to quickly dry shave areas where AED pads will be attached. Wipe away any blood before attaching pads.
4. Stick AED pads to patient.
5. Do not remove AED pads even if the patient has no shockable rhythm or the patient regains a pulse.

If the AED detects a shockable rhythm, if will tell you to stand back before it delivers the shock. After the shock is delivered, immediately resume CPR with chest compressions without checking for a pulse (it takes time before a pulse is able to be felt after defibrillation); check for a pulse 2 minutes after defibrillation. If there is no pulse, check the patient for a shockable rhythm again.

If the patient is in cardiac arrest and no electrical activity is detected (asystole), the AED will inform you that there is "No Shockable Rhythm" and that you will need to continue with manual chest compressions. After 2 minutes of CPR, check the patient for a shockable rhythm again.

Hemorrhaging

Hemorrhaging (severe bleeding) can be internal or external. Signs of internal bleeding include pain, shock, vomiting or coughing blood, loss of consciousness, etc.
- Try to keep the patient calm, warm, and flat.
- Do not remove any objects that have pierced or stabbed the person.
- Put a sterile dressing over the wound. Do not remove the dressing; apply more dressing on top as needed.
- Apply direct pressure to the wound until bleeding stops.
- Once bleeding stops, tape the dressing in place.

Shock

Shock occurs when the body is unable to circulate enough blood to keep organs and tissues functioning properly. It can happen whenever a person is very ill or severely injured. Signs and symptoms of shock include:
- Low or falling blood pressure.
- Rapid and weak pulse.
- Rapid and/or shallow breathing.
- Cold, clammy, pale skin.
- Nausea and vomiting
- Confusion and changes in consciousness

Shock is a severe life threatening condition; immediately call emergency medical services.

Anaphylactic Shock

Anaphylaxis is a severe and life-threatening response to an allergen. Signs and symptoms include:
- Hives and/or rashes
- Wheezing or trouble breathing
- Tongue and/or facial swelling
- Signs and symptoms of shock

Anaphylactic shock is a medical emergency and emergency medical services should be called. If a person has an Epipen (epinephrine), inject the drug into the outer thigh.

Strokes

Strokes occur when blood flow to the brains is prevented, causing brain tissue damage.
Signs and symptoms of a stroke include:

- Weakness/numbness in the face and/or limbs, particularly on only one side of the body.
- Facial drooping or drooling
- Difficulty speaking or understanding
- Nausea/vomiting
- Lost or dimmed vision
- Loss of balance
- Severe headache with sudden onset

Since most effective stroke treatment must be given within 3 hours of symptoms, contact emergency medical services immediately and let them know when symptoms began.

Seizures

A seizure is caused by abnormal electrical activity in the brain resulting in uncontrollable muscle spasms and abnormal consciousness. The most common type of seizure in adults are generalized seizures and symptoms include loss of consciousness, full body convulsions, muscle rigidity, tachycardia, sweating, and hyperventilation. A common type of seizure in children is a febrile seizure; it's typically caused by a high fever and results in loss of consciousness, convulsions, and muscle rigidity. Prolonged seizures (greater than 10 minutes) or recurring seizures without a period of responsiveness indicates the patient is in status epilepticus; status epilepticus is an extreme medical emergency.

- Lower a patient to the floor to prevent falls.
- Place something soft under the patient's head to prevent the head from striking the floor.
- Turn the patient in their side; make sure the head is turned to the side.
- Do not put anything in the patient's mouth.
- Do not try to stop or control the patient's movements.

Concussions

Concussions are brain injuries caused by a blow to the head or any injury that stretches or tears brain tissue. Concussion effects usually appear immediately (altered mental status, nausea, amnesia) or soon after impact and then slowly disappear. In addition to contacting emergency medical services:

- Do not apply direct pressure to the skull if the skull may have been fractured.
- Keep the head, neck, and body aligned.
- Logroll the patient onto their side if they are vomiting.

Fainting

If a person feels faint:

- Have them sit with head between the knees or lie down with legs raised.

If a person has fainted:
- Have them continue to lie down and raise their legs about 12 inches.
- Once they feel better, help them to a sitting position slowly.

Poisoning

Call the Poison Control Center if a person is exhibiting signs and symptoms of poisoning.

Signs and symptoms of poisoning include:
- Burns or redness around the mouth
- Chemical odor
- Vomiting, trouble breathing, confusion
- Burns or stains on clothing or person
- Empty drug bottles or spilled drugs

If poison gets in a person's eyes or skin, remove glasses, contact lenses, or clothing and rinse with water for 15 to 20 minutes.

If a person inhaled poison, move them to an area with fresh air.

If a person swallowed poison, do not induce vomiting or give them anything to eat or drink unless directed by the Poison Control Center.

Concussions

Concussions are caused by blows to the head or any event that causes the head to move back and forth quickly. They can be minor or life-threatening. Signs of a serious concussion include:
- Headache that worsens or won't go away
- Stiff neck
- Weakness or loss of coordination
- Slurred speech
- Very sleepy or hard to awaken
- One pupil is larger than the other
- Convulsions or seizures
- Confusion or unusual behavior
- Loss of consciousness

Emergency care includes:
- Activating the EMS system
- Placing hands on both sides of the head to keep it aligned with the spine.
- Do not apply pressure to the skull if the skull may be fractured.
- Logroll the person onto the side if they are vomiting.

Burns

Burn injuries can affect more than just the skin. They can cause fluid loss, swelling of the airways, and damage the nerve endings. The severity of burns depends on the depth of the burn, amount of body area affected, whether burns were to critical areas of the body, associated trauma/pre-existing medical conditions, and age of patient. Burns to the respiratory tract, face, hands, feet, genitalia are more serious. Those with associated trauma or preexisting conditions or are younger than 5 or greater than 55 may have a harder time healing from a burn injury. Severe burns can lead to sepsis, hypothermia, shock and respiratory distress.

First degree/superficial burns: affects the epidermis only; painful and red, but no blisters.
Second degree/partial thickness burns: affects the epidermis and parts of dermis, painful, red, and blisters.
Third degree/full thickness burns: affects entire dermis and there is no pain; skin may appear white and waxy or black and charred.

Contact emergency medical services for severe burns.
- Do not touch the person if they are in contact with an electrical source. Turn off electrical source before touching patient.
- Do not apply any ointments to burned areas as that could cause heat retention.
- Remove patient from the source of the burn and flush the affected area with water or saline; do not immerse the area. If the patient has third degree burns, unless the patient is on fire, do not flush them with water as they are at risk for hypothermia.
- Remove any clothing unless clothing is clinging to the skin.
- Cover burned area with dressing. Check local protocols regarding whether to use moist or dry dressing; moist dressing can lead to hypothermia.
- Keep patient warm since burn injuries may damage the body's temperature regulation system.

Assisting with Physical Exams

Physical exams are conducted by nurses or doctors; nursing assistants may assist. Consent must be given before an exam is conducted.

Babies, toddlers, and school-age children are undressed, with diapers and underpants left on. Diapers and underpants are removed as needed. Parents are present when children are examined.

Always practice hand hygiene before and after the exam and provide for patient privacy. Stay in the exam room if:
- You are female, the patient is female, and the examiner is male
- You are male, the patient is male, and the examiner is male
- You are male and the female examiner wants you there when examining a male

1. Tell the patient what clothing to remove and have them put on a gown.
2. Ask the patient to void; collect a urine specimen if needed.
3. Measure and record the patient's vital signs, weight, and height.
4. Position and drape the patient as directed.
    a. Dorsal recumbent position: the patient is in a supine position with their legs open; used to examine the abdomen, chest, breasts; knees are raised and legs spread to examine the perineal area
    b. Lithotomy position: the patient is in a supine position with knees raised, hips at the edge of the table, and legs spread; used to examine the vagina and cervix
    c. Knee-chest position: the patient is in a prone position with their body resting on their knees and chest; the arms are extended and the abdomen raised; used to examine the anal area
    d. Sim's position: sometimes used to examine the anal and genital areas
5. Place a waterproof pad under the buttocks.
6. Put the call light on for the examiner.
7. After the exam:
    a. Discard disposable items and clean reusable items
    b. Return items to the tray or storage area; replace supplies on the exam tray
    c. Put clean drawsheet or paper on exam table
    d. Label specimens and take them to the correct area

Collecting Specimens

Never touch the inside of a specimen container to prevent contaminating the container.

Routine Urine Specimen

1. Attach the label with patient information to the specimen container. Attach a "biohazard" label to the transport bag.
2. Practice hand hygiene and put on gloves.
3. Ask the patient to urinate into a bedpan, urinal, or specimen collection pan (hat). Secure the urinal cap before taking the urinal to the bathroom.
4. Pour 120 mL of urine into the specimen container or fill the specimen container three quarters full.
5. Place a lid on the specimen container. Remove and discard one glove. Use the ungloved hand to hold the transport bag and the gloved hand to put the container into the bag. Do not touch the outside of the transport bag with your gloved hand to prevent contaminating it.
6. Remove other glove, perform hand hygiene, and put on new gloves.
7. Clean and disinfect equipment used.
8. Remove and discard gloves. Practice hand hygiene.
9. Take specimen to designated area.

Clean Catch (Midstream) Urine Specimen

1. Attach the label with patient information to the specimen container. Attach a "biohazard" label to the transport bag.
2. Practice hand hygiene and put on gloves.
3. Clean the patient's perineal area.
4. If the patient is female, have her hold the labia open until the urine specimen is collected. If the patient is an uncircumcised male, have him keep the foreskin pulled back until the urine specimen is collected.
5. Ask the patient to start urinating into a bedpan, urinal, or hat. Tell them to stop urinating. If the patient cannot stop urinating, pass the specimen container into the urine stream.
6. Hold the specimen container under the patient and ask them to continue urinating. Collect at least 30 mL of urine.
7. Place a lid on the specimen container. Remove and discard one glove. Use the ungloved hand to hold the transport bag and the gloved hand to put the container into the bag. Do not touch the outside of the transport bag with your gloved hand to prevent contaminating it.
8. Remove other glove, perform hand hygiene, and put on new gloves.
9. Clean and disinfect equipment used.
10. Remove and discard gloves. Practice hand hygiene.
11. Take specimen to designated area.

Collecting a Stool Specimen

1. Attach the label with patient information to the specimen container. Attach a "biohazard" label to the transport bag.
2. Practice hand hygiene and put on gloves.
3. Ask the patient to empty into a bedpan or hat. Tell them not to throw toilet paper into the bedpan or hat; provide a disposable bag for them to dispose soiled tissues.
4. When the patient is finished, provide perineal care if needed.
5. Use a tongue depressor to transfer 1 to 2 tablespoons of stool to the specimen container. Take the sample from:
   a. Middle of a stool
   b. Areas of pus, mucus, or bloody and watery areas
   c. Middle and both ends of a hard stool
6. Wrap the tongue depressor with toilet paper and discard it in the disposable bag.
7. Place a lid on the specimen container. Remove and discard one glove. Use the ungloved hand to hold the transport bag and the gloved hand to put the container into the bag. Do not touch the outside of the transport bag with your gloved hand to prevent contaminating it.
8. Remove other glove, perform hand hygiene, and put on new gloves.
9. Clean and disinfect equipment used.
10. Remove and discard gloves. Practice hand hygiene.
11. Take specimen to designated area.

Collection a 24 Hour Urine Specimen

During a 24 hour urine specimen collection, the patient voids to start the test with an empty bladder; this voiding is discarded. All voidings in the next 24 hours are saved; the test has to be restarted if any voiding was not saved, toilet tissue was thrown into the specimen, or the specimen contains stool. The patient is asked to do a final voiding at the end of the 24 hour period. The collected urine is chilled or refrigerated to prevent growth of bacteria; a preservative may also be added to the collection container.

1. Practice hand hygiene and put on gloves.
2. Ask the patient to void. Measure and discard the urine. Write the time on the urine container as this marks the start of the 24 hour period.
3. Remove gloves and practice hand hygiene.
4. Mark the test start and end times on the room and bathroom labels.
5. Do the following every time the patient voids:
   a. Remind them to not have a bowel movement when voiding, use the voiding device, discard tissues in toilet or wastebasket, and put on call light after voiding.
   b. Practice hand hygiene and put on gloves.
   c. Measure urine and pour urine into the urine container.
   d. Remove gloves, perform hand hygiene, and put on new gloves.

e. Clean and disinfect equipment.

f. Remove gloves and perform hand hygiene.

Collecting a Urine Specimen From an Infant or Child

1. Practice hand hygiene and put on gloves.
2. Put the patient on their back and remove diapers.
3. Clean the perineal area with cotton balls.
4. Remove gloves, practice hand hygiene, and put on new gloves.
5. Remove adhesive backing from the collection bag. Spread the patient's legs and apply the bag to the perineum area.
6. Cut a slit in the bottom of a new diaper, put the diaper on the child, and pull the collection bag through the diaper slit.
7. Remove gloves and practice hand hygiene.
8. Once the patient has voided:
   a. Attach label with patient information to the specimen container. Attach a "biohazard" label to the transport bag.
   b. Practice hand hygiene and put on gloves.
   c. Remove the diaper and collection bag.
   d. Seal the collection bag or transfer the urine to the specimen container using the drainage tab.
   e. Clean the perineal area and put diapers on the patient.
   f. Remove gloves and practice hand hygiene.

Collecting a Sputum Specimen

1. Practice hand hygiene and put on gloves.
2. Attach the label to the specimen container.
3. Have the patient rinse their mouth with water to clean the mouth. Do not use mouthwash as mouthwash can kill bacteria, resulting in accurate test results.
4. Tell the patient to cough deeply for the sputum. The sputum for analysis should come from the lungs because that is where most of the microbes are.
5. Have the patient spit the sputum into the specimen container and close the lid.
6. Remove gloves and practice hand hygiene.

Blood Glucose Testing

A glucometer is used to measure blood glucose levels, often used for diabetic patients. Try to select a good site for a skin puncture:

- Avoid areas with calluses because those areas have poor blood flow (e.g., thumbs and index fingers)
- Avoid swollen, bruised, scarred, or cyanotic areas
- Do not use sites with many nerve endings which can make it painful (e.g., center or fleshy parts of fingers)
- Use the side of the middle or ring finger tip

1. Practice hand hygiene and put on gloves.
2. Wipe the glucometer with an antiseptic wipe.
3. Follow manufacturer instructions for turning on and operating the glucometer. Insert a test strip into the glucometer.
4. Select a skin puncture site and increase blood flow to the puncture site by rubbing the site gently or applying a warm washcloth.
5. Wipe the site with an antiseptic wipe and let it dry.
6. Puncture the skin with the lancet and let a large drop of blood form.
7. Dip the test strip into the drop of blood. The glucometer will test the sample when there is enough blood on the strip.
8. Use a gauze to apply pressure to the puncture site to stop the bleeding.
9. Read the result on the glucometer display and record.
10. Discard the lancet in sharps container.
11. Discard the gauze and test strip according to facility policy.
12. Remove gloves and practice hand hygiene.

Wound Care

Wounds may be open or closed. An open wound is any break in the skin or mucous membrane. A closed wound is when tissues are injured, but the skin is intact. Examples of closed wounds include bruises (contusions), sprains, etc. Examples of open wounds include:

- abrasion: caused by the scraping of the skin surface by friction; keep clean and dry to prevent infection
- laceration: caused by the tearing of body tissue
- excoriation: loss of top layer of skin due to scratching or rubbing
- puncture/penetrating wounds: caused by sharp pointed objects
- avulsion: occurs when a body part is torn away by trauma or surgery; it can range from minor (skin flaps) to moderate (degloving) to severe (amputation);
- degloving injury: occurs when soft tissue, down to the bone, is stripped off the body part; this most often happens to appendages, but can happen to the scalp when hair is caught in machinery
- amputation: the complete or partial loss of a limb
- evisceration: when internal organs of the body are pushed outside the body
- ulcer: an open sore on the skin or mucous membrane

Ulcers

Venous ulcers are open sores caused by bad venous blood flow. They are typically found on the lower legs or feet, inner parts of the ankles, and heels. Arterial ulcers are open sores caused by bad arterial blood flow. They are typically found on the lower legs or feet, between toes, top of toes, and outer side of the ankle.

Pressure Ulcers (Bedsores)

Pressure ulcers are caused by prolonged pressure on the skin that decreases blood supply to the area, resulting in a skin sore. It may also be caused by friction and shearing. They are typically found over bony body parts such as the tailbone, hip, back, elbow, spines, shoulder, side or back of heads, etc. Patients that can't walk, have poor nutrition, have poor circulation, or have trouble healing are at higher risk for developing pressure ulcers. The "Braden" scale is used by licensed nurses to determine a patient's risk of developing a pressure ulcer.

Pressure ulcers are staged as follows:
- Stage 1: Skin appears red (pale, blue, or purple in those with dark skin) and is intact. The color does not fade with pressure.
- Stage 2: There may be a shallow crater or a blister (intact or open).
- Stage 3: The skin (epidermis and dermis layer) is gone and subcutaneous fat may be exposed.
- Stage 4: The muscle, tendon, and/or bone may be exposed.
- Unstageable: The skin and subcutaneous tissue are gone. The ulcer is covered by slough (soft, moist, light-colored dead tissue) or eschar (tough, dry, dark-colored dead

tissue). The stage (typically, stage 3 or 4) cannot be determined until all the slough and eschar are removed.

- Suspected deep tissue injury: Skin appears purple or maroon and is intact. There may be a blood filled blister. This type of injury may be difficult to detect in those with dark skin.

Protective devices to prevent pressure ulcers:
- A bed cradle is placed over a person and beneath top linens to prevent pressure on the legs, feet, and toes.
- Have patients wear heel and elbow protectors to reduce shear and friction.
- Use gel or fluid-filled pads or cushions for chairs and wheelchairs.
- Air-fluidized beds keep a patient's body weight distributed evenly and relieves pressure on bony areas.
- Alternating pressure beds have areas that inflate and deflate on a rotating basis, shifting the pressure from one area to another.

To help prevent ulcers:
- Reposition patients at least every 2 hours
- Avoid tight clothing
- Tell patients to not sit with their legs crossed
- Do not scrub or rub the skin
- Avoid pressure on the heels of feet and other bony areas
- Wear well fitting shoes and break in new shoes slowly
- Use proper protective devices

Wound Dressings

The doctors and nurses will choose what types of dressings to use. Dressings are applied to wounds to protect wounds from further injury and microbes, absorb drainage, control bleeding with pressure, and provide a moist environment for wound healing. Dressings may be dry or wet. In dry dressings, the wound is covered with a dry gauze. In wet dressings, the wound is covered with a wet dressing and then covered with dry dressing.

Dressings must be secured to prevent microbes from entering the wound and to prevent drainage from leaking. Tapes and Montgomery ties are used to secure dressings. Apply tape to the top, middle, and bottom of a dressing, with the tape extending several inches beyond the side of the dressing. Do not encircle a body part with tape as that can cut off circulation if swelling occurs. Tape is removed by pulling it towards the wound. Montgomery ties are used to secure larger dressings and/or dressings that require frequent changes. In Montgomery ties, the adhesive strips are placed on the sides of the wound and the cloth ties are tied over the dressing. The adhesive strips remain while the cloth ties are undone during dressing changes.

Common types of dressings include:

- Gauze: absorbs drainage
- Non-adherent gauze: gauze with a non-stick surface to prevent sticking to the wound
- Transparent adhesive film: allows air, but not microbes to reach the wound; drainage is NOT absorbed; allows for wound observation

Applying a Dry, Non-Sterile Dressing

1. Practice hand hygiene and put on gloves.
2. Remove tape or untie Montgomery ties.
   a. If removing tape, pull tape towards the wound.
   b. If undoing Montgomery ties, fold ties away from the wound.
3. Using forceps, wet a gauze with adhesive remover and remove any adhesive from the skin, wiping away from the wound.
4. Using forceps, remove the old gauze dressings from the wound and place them in a plastic bag; do not let the patient see the soiled dressing and do not let the gauze touch the outside of the bag. If the dressing is stuck to the wound, moisten the dressing with a saline solution.
5. Observe and make note of wound appearance and drainage.
6. Remove gloves, practice hand hygiene, and put on new gloves.
7. Open the new dressing package.
8. Using forceps, clean the wound with saline.
   a. Clean the wound, starting from top to bottom and stroking from the wound to the surrounding skin.
   b. Use a clean gauze for each stroke.
9. Apply and secure dressings as directed by the nurse.
10. Remove gloves and practice hand hygiene.

Wound Drainage

There are 4 common types of wound drainage:
- Serous drainage: clear, watery fluid; fluid in a blister is serous
- Sanguineous drainage: bloody drainage; bright red drainage indicates newer bleeding whereas dark red drainage indicates older bleeding
- Serosanguineous drainage: thin, watery drainage that is red tinged
- Purulent drainage: thick green, yellow, or brown drainage

Some patients may have a drain at the wound site; this is done when a large amount of drainage is expected. The amount and kind of wound drainage should be observed and measured.

There are 3 ways to measure wound drainage:
- Weigh dressings before applying them and after removing them; the difference is the weight of the drainage
- Note the number and size of dressings with drainage
- For closed drainages, measure the amount of drainage in the container

Prepping For Surgery

Pre-Operative Care

As part of pre-operative care, patients are emotionally prepped for surgery. To reduce a patient's anxiety, the health care team will go over the following with the patient:
- Explanation of why surgery is needed and the benefits and risks of surgery
- What to expect during the recovery period
- Explain the pre and post operative procedures
- The purposes of any medications or tests
- Any concerns the patient may have

Patients are usually put on NPO status for 6 to 8 hours before surgery; this is done to prevent vomiting and aspiration. Remove cups and water pitchers from the room and remind patients and their family that NPO means nothing by mouth, including water, ice, gum, and mints.

During the morning of surgery, the nurse may ask you to help with the following:
- Administering a cleansing enema or vaginal douche to clear the bowels or vaginal canal.
- A complete bath to reduce microbes. A special cleanser and shampoo may be ordered.
- Removing makeup, nail polish, and fake nails because the skin, lips, and nail beds are observed for color and circulation during surgery.
- Remove wigs, hair clips, etc. A surgical cap keeps hair off the face.
- Remove jewelry, rings, etc. because fingers can swell during surgery.
- Remove dentures because they can be a choking hazard during surgery. Allow the patient to wear dentures as long as possible.
- Remove prosthetic devices, contact lenses, hearing aids, etc. Hearing aids may be left in if the surgeon needs to talk to the patient during surgery.

To reduce the risk of infection, a skin prep is done before surgery. Skin prep usually involves cleansing the area with anti-microbial soap and trimming or removing hair around the surgical site. A skin prep kit is used for shaving.

1. Practice hand hygiene and put on gloves.
2. Adjust the bed to a comfortable working height, lock the wheels, and lower the side rail on the side you are working on.
3. Cover the patient with a bath blanket, fan-fold top linens to the bottom of the bed, and place a waterproof pad under the area to be shaved.
4. Open the skin prep skit.
5. Position and drape the patient.
6. Lather the skin with the sponge.
7. Hold the skin taut and shave in the direction of growth and outward from the center.
8. Check for cuts, nicks, and scratches.

9. Rinse and pat dry the skin.
10. Remove the drape and waterproof pad.
11. Remove gloves and practice hand hygiene.
12. Bring the top linens back up and remove the bath blanket.

Post-Operative Care

After surgery, the patient is taken to the post-anesthesia care unit (PACU). While the patient is in surgery or recovery, prepare the patient's room. Once the PACU nurses transfer the patient to the patient's room, help them transfer the patient to the bed. You will be responsible for measuring vital signs and observing the patient.

The nurse will tell you how often to measure the patient's vital signs, which is typically:
- Every 15 minutes until the patient is stable
- Every 30 minutes for 1 to 2 hours
- Every hour for 4 hours
- Then every 4 hours

The patient will be positioned to promote easy breathing, prevent stress on incision sites, and prevent aspiration. They are repositioned every 1 to 2 hours to prevent respiratory and circulatory issues.

Observe the patient for the following signs and alert the nurse:
- Abdominal distention, pain, and/or cramping
- Anxiety
- Bleeding
- Changes in blood pressure
- Chest pain
- Confusion, disorientation, changes in mental state
- Weak cough
- Changes in respiration
- Drainage from wounds or dressing
- Moist, pale, or clammy skin
- Urinary issues
- Nausea, vomiting
- The patient must void within 8 hours of surgery; if they do not, a catheter may be required.

Preventing Respiratory Complications

Older patients are at higher risk for respiratory complications due to having weaker respiratory muscles and less elastic lung tissue. Have patients practice coughing and deep breathing exercise, and incentive spirometry to prevent respiratory complications such as pneumonia and atelectasis. To promote comfort, have patients hold a pillow or their hand over their incision site when coughing.

Preventing Circulatory Complications

When patients are sedentary, blood flow slows down and blood clots may form and lead to pulmonary embolisms. To increase blood flow:
- Perform leg exercises
- Encourage the patient to walk as soon as possible
- Wear elastic stockings; elastic stockings put pressure on the veins, returning blood to the heart
- Use sequential compression devices

The nurse will tell you when to do the leg exercises; typically, every 1 or 2 hours while a patient is awake. To perform leg exercises, have the patient:
- Rotate their ankles
- Make circles with their toes
- Flex the feet
- Bend and extend each knee
- Raise and lower each leg off the bed

When applying elastic stockings, make sure you use the correct size; the nurse will tell you what size to use. The toe opening should be over the top of the toes or under the toes; the toe opening is used to check skin color, circulation, and temperature. Elastic stockings are usually worn for 30 minutes every 8 hours. Elastic bandages may be used in place of elastic stockings.

When applying elastic bandages:
1. Hold the bandage so that the roll is up and the loose end is at the bottom.
2. Make 2 circles around the smallest part of the wrist, foot, ankle, or knee.
3. Make upward and overlapping spirals.
4. Make 2 circles at the end and secure the bandage with Velcro, tape, or clips.
5. Check the fingers and/or toes for skin color, circulation, and temperature.

Skill: Applying Elastic Stockings
1. Have the patient lie in the supine position.
2. Adjust the bed height to a comfortable working position.
3. Turn stockings inside out, at least to the heel.
4. Place the foot of the stocking over the toes, foot, and heel.
5. Pull the top of stocking over the foot, heel, and leg. Avoid forcing or over-extending any part of the leg.
6. **Ensure that there are no twists or wrinkles. The heel of the stocking should be over the heel and the opening in the toe area, if present, should be over or under the toe area.**
7. Return the bed to the low position.

8. Wash your hands.

Caring For The Terminally Ill

Patients have a right to make end of life decision, including the right to refuse medical treatment. They may have a "Do Not Resuscitate" order and/or an advance directive, such as a living will. Both "Do Not Resuscitate" orders and advance directives are legally binding documents. In an advance directive, the patient may detail allowances and restrictions for treatment should they become terminally ill; they may also give someone else "power of attorney" to make decisions for them should they become incapacitated. "Do Not Resuscitate" orders only go into effect when a patient goes into respiratory or cardiac arrest; they should be provided life-saving treatment unless they go into respiratory or cardiac arrest.

Terminally ill patients may choose palliative care or hospice care. Both palliative and hospice care revolve around making a patient comfortable, not curing the patient. The difference between the two is that palliative care can be given at the same time as treatments meant to cure the illness, whereas hospice care is generally started after treatment for the disease has stopped and it is clear the patient will die.

Stages of Grief/Dying

1. Denial
2. Anger (Why me?)
3. Bargaining.
4. Depression
5. Acceptance

Not everyone goes through all the stages of grief, nor do they go through the stages in order.

Providing Care

- Report signs and symptoms of pain immediately.
- Hearing is the last function to go, so provide words of comfort and explanations about care.
- As dying patients lose their appetite, do not force patients to eat, but notify the nurse.
- Body temperatures may rise even though the skin feels cool, provide light covering as blankets may be too warm. Observe for signs the patient is cold.

Signs Of Impending Death

Signs of impending death include Cheyne-Stokes respirations (rapid, irregular, and shallow breathing followed by decreased breathing and periods of no breathing); decreased blood pressure; rapid, weak pulse; cold and blue lips, hands, feets; decreased body movement, functions and awareness.

Assisting with Port Mortem Care

Rigor mortis is the stiffening of joints and muscles after death; the patient's body is put in normal alignment before rigor mortis sets in. You may expect to hear sounds when you move the body as air is expelled.

1. Wash hands and collect post-mortem kit, bed-linen protector, towels and washcloths, bath basin, denture cup, tape, cotton balls, and valuables envelope.
2. Put on gloves and put the patient in a supine position.
3. Close the eyes; put moist cotton balls over the eyelids if the eyes will not stay close.
4. Follow agency policy regarding denture care.
5. Close the patient's mouth; if necessary, keep the mouth closed by putting a rolled towel under the chin.
6. Follow agency policy regarding jewelry removal. Put jewelry in a valuables envelope.
7. Unless an autopsy is ordered, remove all drainage bags, tubes, and catheters.
8. Wash, and dry, soiled areas with plain water.
9. Put a waterproof pad under the buttocks.
10. Replace soiled dressings with clean ones.
11. Put a clean gown on the patient.
12. Brush/comb the hair if necessary.
13. Cover the patient with a clean sheet, up to shoulder level.
14. Put the patient's personal belongings in a bag, labelled with their name.
15. Tidy up the room and allow the family to view the body.
16. After the family has viewed the body, fill out ID tags and place one on the ankle and the other on the opposite big toe.
17. Place the body in the shroud and attach an ID tag to the shroud.
18. Pull the privacy curtain around the bed and close the door.
19. Record and report time the body was taken to funeral director and what was done with valuables and dentures.

Data Collection and Reporting

Daily observation of patients can provide clues into their physical and mental health. Signs are things you can observe (see, touch, smell, hear) such as vomiting, wheezing, etc. Symptoms are things only the patient can tell you such as nausea, pain, etc. Objective data is data you observed; subjective data is data that the patient tells you. Subjective data is just as important as objective data. When reporting changes and observations, use as much of the patient's own words as possible.

A patient's records/charts are considered medical records and are legal documents. When documenting your observations:

- Use black or blue ink.
- Sign your name and title to all entries.
- Never erase or use liquid eraser to correct mistakes; always cross it out with a line and write your initials next to it.
- Be objective and never record your opinions.
- Use quotes when including what patients tell you.
- Use the 24 hour clock when recording time.

Activities of Daily Living

As people age, they may experience age related changes such as the following:
- Reduction in immunity (the ability to fight off disease)
- Increased risk for chronic illnesses. Chronic illnesses such as dementia, Alzheimer's, circulatory diseases, stroke, etc. can affect thinking and reasoning.
- Reduced muscle strength, flexibility, and stability
- Decreased vision and hearing
- Decreased ability to sense pain
- Changes in sleep habits
- Reduced short term memory, word recall, and abstract thinking
- Increased chance of falling (falls are a leading cause of death in the elderly)

Allow patients to be involved in their activities of daily living (personal care, grooming, etc.) to promote self control and independence.

Hygiene

It is important that you help patients practice good hygiene to help patients feel clean and prevent disease. Early morning care (AM care) is done before breakfast. Morning care is done after breakfast. Evening care (PM care) is done at bedtime.

During AM care, wash patients' face and teeth and/or dentures; assist with elimination; assist with dressing and hair care; assist patient with breakfast.

During PM care, assist with elimination; assist patients with oral hygiene and face washing; help patients change into pajamas; prepare patients for sleep; may include a massage or other activity to help patients relax.

Bathing

Follow the bathing schedule in a patient's care plan. Due to older patients having drier skin, they are often not given daily complete baths; instead, they may be given daily partial paths. When bathing patients, ensure their privacy and safety. Use assistive devices to secure patients that are at high risk of falls; however, only use assistive devices as authorized by facility policies, unauthorized usage could be considered a restraint.

Bathing guidelines:
- Always check with the care plan to ensure that the patient is allowed to have a bath
- Ensure water temperature is safe.
- Bathing stimulates the need to urinate so it's best to have the patient urinate before giving a bath.

- Wash the body from the cleanest area to the dirtiest area; front to back and top to bottom. Always used a clean part of the washcloth for each stroke.
- Squeeze out excess water every time you change washcloths. Put used washcloths in the laundry bag; do not put used washcloths back in the water basin.
- Do not let bath towels, shower spray or other bathing equipment touch the floor.
- Disinfect the tub and shower equipment after the bath.
- If a patient becomes weak or faints during bathing, stop the bathing process, stay with the resident (do not leave them in the bath), and call for assistance; immediately report the incident to the licensed nurse.
- Record and report the bathing activity.

The many benefits of bathing include:
- Keeps patients clean.
- Improves circulation by stimulating the muscles.
- Provides exercise for the joints and limbs.
- Gives CNAs the opportunity to inspect the patient's skin, mobility, and health.

Tub Baths

Tub baths should not last longer than 20 minutes; tub baths can make patients feel weak, tired, or faint. Wash the upper body, between skin folds, under breasts, and perineal area. Pat the patient dry.

Showers

If the shower does not have a non-skid surface, a bath mat must be used. Patients that can't stand can use:
- Shower chairs: a patient can sit in a shower chair during a shower; the shower chair contains openings from which water drains. Lock the chair during the shower and use the chair to transport the patient to and from the shower.
- Shower stalls/cabinets: a person can be wheeled into shower stalls/cabinets; a hand held nozzle is available to give the shower.
- Shower trolleys (portable tubs): transfer a patient from the bed to the shower trolley; with the patient lying down, use the available hand held nozzle to give the shower.

Skill: Provide Female Perineal Care

1. Perform hand hygiene and put on gloves.
2. Adjust the bed to a comfortable working level and lock the wheels.
3. Lower the head of the bed so it's as flat as possible or as flat as the patient can tolerate. The patient should be lying on her back.
4. Fill a wash basin with warm water (110F to 115F). Add no-rinse cleansing solution if being used. Ask the patient to check the water temperature.
5. Lower the side rail on the side you will be working from. Raise the side rail on the opposite side.

6. Cover the patient with a bath blanket and remove top linens to the foot of the bed.
7. Help the patient undress.
8. Help the patient bend her knees and spread her legs to expose the perineal area (only exposing area between hip and knees); if the patient cannot spread her legs enough to expose the perineal area, turn the patient on her side with the knees bent forward to expose the perineal area.
9. Position the bath blanket like a diamond; so that one corner is at the neck and 1 corner is between the legs. Wrap one corner under and around each leg.
10. Put a bed protector under the patient's buttocks to keep the bed dry.
11. Lift the corner of the blanket that is between the legs, to expose the perineal area.
12. Wet a washcloth. Make a mitt with the washcloth. Always wash with a clean area of the washcloth. Apply soap or no-rinse solution to the washcloth.
13. **Clean the vaginal area. Always use a clean part of the washcloth for each stroke.**
    a. **Separate the labia.**
    b. **Clean 1 side of the labia from front to back (top to bottom).**
    c. **Repeat on other side of the labia.**
    d. **Clean from the top of the vulva and stroking down to to the anus.**
    e. **Rinse and dry the vaginal area.**
14. Turn the patient so that they are facing away from you. Adjust the bath blankets so that only the buttocks are exposed.
15. Wet a washcloth. Make a mitt with the washcloth. Apply soap or no-rinse solution to the washcloth.
16. Separate the buttocks and wash from the vagina to the back. Clean one side, then the other side, and then the middle. Rinse and dry.
17. Reposition the patient.
18. Empty, rinse, and dry the basin. Put the basin in the dirty supply area.
19. Remove the bed protector.
20. Remove and discard gloves. Practice hand hygiene and put on clean gloves.
21. Provide clean linens and incontinence products as needed.
22. Remove gloves and wash hands.
23. Report and record any observations.

Male Perineal Care

1. Perform hand hygiene and put on gloves.
2. Adjust the bed to a comfortable working level and lock the wheels.
3. Lower the head of the bed so it's as flat as possible or as flat as the patient can tolerate. The patient should be lying on his back.
4. Fill a wash basin with warm water (110F to 115F). Add no-rinse cleansing solution if being used. Ask the patient to check the water temperature.
5. Lower the side rail on the side you will be working from. Raise the side rail on the opposite side.
6. Cover the patient with a bath blanket and remove top linens to the foot of the bed.
7. Help the patient undress.

8. Help the patient bend his knees and spread his legs to expose the perineal area; if the patient cannot spread his legs enough to expose the perineal area, turn the patient on his side with the knees bent forward to expose the perineal area.
9. Position the bath blanket like a diamond; so that one corner is at the neck and 1 corner is between the legs. Wrap one corner under and around each leg.
10. Put a bed protector under the patient's buttocks to keep the bed dry.
11. Lift the corner of the blanket that is between the legs, to expose the perineal area.
12. Wet a washcloth. Make a mitt with the washcloth. Always wash with a clean area of the washcloth. Apply soap or no-rinse solution to the washcloth.
13. If the patient is uncircumcised, retract the foreskin.
14. Hold the penis and clean from the tip down to the base of the penis, using circular motions. Using a clean washcloth, repeat the same steps to rinse and dry the penis. After rinsing, return the foreskin to its natural position.
15. Wet a washcloth. Make a mitt with the washcloth. Always wash with a clean area of the washcloth. Apply soap or no-rinse solution to the washcloth.
16. Wash the scrotum and perineum. Rinse and dry.
17. Turn the patient so that they are facing away from you. Adjust the bath blankets so that only the buttocks are exposed.
18. Wet a washcloth. Make a mitt with the washcloth. Apply soap or no-rinse solution to the washcloth.
19. Separate the buttocks and wash from the perineum to the back. Clean one side, then the other side, and then the middle. Rinse and dry.
20. Remove the bed protector.
21. Remove and discard gloves. Practice hand hygiene and put on clean gloves.
22. Provide clean linens and incontinence products as needed.
23. Report and record any observations.

Giving Complete Bed Baths

1. Perform hand hygiene and put on gloves.
2. Adjust the bed to a comfortable working level and lock the wheels.
3. Cover the patient with a bath blanket and remove top linens.
4. Help the patient undress.
5. Lower the head of the bed so it's as flat as possible or as flat as the patient can tolerate.
6. Put a pillow under the patient's head.
7. Fill a wash basin with warm water (110F to 115F). Add no-rinse cleansing solution if being used. Ask the patient to check the water temperature.
8. Lower the bed rail on the side you're working on.
9. Place a towel over the patient's chest to keep the bath blanket dry.
10. Make a mitt with the washcloth. Always wash with a clean area of the washcloth.
    a. Wash the eyes without soap; wipe from the inner eye to the outer corner.
11. Ask the patient if they would like to use soap on their face. Rinse the washcloth and apply soap, if requested. Wash the face, neck, and ears. Rinse and pat dry.

12. Place a bed protector or bath towel under the patient's far arm to keep the bed dry. Wash the shoulder, arm, and underarms, using long downward strokes. Put the patient's hand in a basin of water and wash the hand. Rinse and pat dry. Remove the bed protector.
13. Exercise the patient's hand and fingers.
14. Repeat for the other arm.
15. Place a towel over the patient's chest, horizontally. Hold the towel in place and pull the bath blanket down to the waist, from under the towel.
16. Apply soap to the washcloth and wash the patient's chest, under the towel. Do not expose the person. Rinse and pat dry.
17. Hold the towel in place and pull the bath blanket down to the pubic area. Apply soap to the washcloth and wash the patient's abdomen. Rinse and pat dry.
18. Pull the bath blanket back up to the shoulders; the bath blanket should cover both arms. Remove the towel.
19. Change the water in the basin if it's too cool or soapy.
20. Fold the bath blanket so that the far leg is exposed. Place a bed protector or bath towel under the leg. Apply soap to a washcloth and wash the leg, using long downward strokes. Rinse and pat dry.
21. Place foot in the basin of water and wash the foot. Be sure to wash between the toes. Rinse and dry; be sure to dry between the toes as well.
22. Cover the leg with the bath blanket and remove the bed protector or bath towel.
23. Repeat for the other leg and foot.
24. Change the water in the basin if it's too cool or soapy.
25. Turn the person so they are facing away from you. The bath blanket should cover the patient's front (only the back and buttocks should be exposed). Place a bed protector alongside the patient's back.
26. Apply soap to a washcloth and wash the back, starting from the neck and working your way down to the buttocks. Rinse and pat dry. An optional back massage may be given at this point. Remove bed protector and turn the patient onto their back.
27. Change water for perineal care. Practice proper hand hygiene and change gloves.
28. If the patient is able to perform perineal care, allow them to. If not, provide perineal care.
29. Remove gloves and practice proper hand hygiene. Put on new gloves.
30. Apply lotion, deodorant, etc. as requested or ordered.
31. Help the patient dress.
32. Gather soiled linens and towels and place them in the hamper.
33. Remove and dispose gloves.
34. Report and record any observations.

Skill: Giving Modified/Partial Bed Baths

1. Perform hand hygiene and put on gloves.
2. Adjust the bed to a comfortable working level. Lock the wheels.
3. Cover the patient with a bath blanket and remove top linens.
4. Help the patient undress and put garments in soiled linen container.

5. Fill a wash basin with warm water (110F to 115F). Add no-rinse cleansing solution if being used. Ask the patient to check the water temperature.
6. Wash hands and put on clean gloves
7. Position the patient in Fowler's position or have them sit at the bedside.
8. The face, hands, underarms, backs, buttocks, and perineal area are washed for a partial bath.
9. **Beginning with the eyes, wash eyes with a wet washcloth (no soap) from the inner eye to outer eye. Use a clean area of the washcloth for each stroke. Wash the face.**
10. Dry the patient's face with a dry cloth.
11. Expose one arm. Place a bed protector or bath towel under the patient's arm to keep the bed dry.
12. Apply soap to a wet washcloth. Wash fingers, underneath fingernails, hand, arm, and underarm, keeping the rest of the body covered. Rinse and pat dry.
13. See "*Giving Complete Bed Baths*" section for instructions on how to wash other parts of the body.
14. Remove and discard gloves. Practice proper hand hygiene and put on new gloves.
15. Give an optional back massage.
16. Apply lotion, deodorant, etc. as requested or ordered.
17. Help the patient dress.
18. Remove and dispose gloves.
19. Report and record any observations.

Skin Care

- Only licensed nurses can apply prescription ointments, lotions, etc. to a patient's skin.
- Observe patients skin for any sores, redness, or abnormalities that could indicate disease and report it to the licensed nurse.
- Keep skin free of pressure; pressure can lead to pressure ulcers (bedsores).
- Keep skin dry in the axilla (underarms), beneath the breasts, genitals, perineum, buttocks, and other skin creases to prevent bacterial growth.
- Avoid talcs or powders that can cake between skin folds.

Oral Care

You may need to brush a patient's teeth or dentures and keep their mouth moist and free of debris; a dry mouth leads to bad breath and increases the risk for tooth decay and skin breakage. Bad oral hygiene may also increase the risk of periodontal disease (gum disease). In order to keep a patient's mouth moist, you may need to provide oral care every hour or two. If a patient is unconscious, they will require more frequent oral care to keep their mouth moist.

Skill: Provide Mouth Care
1. Have the patient sit at a 75 to 90 degree angle
2. Place a towel across the patient's chest to protect the patient's clothing.
3. Perform hand hygiene and put on gloves.
4. Moisten toothbrush with water and then apply toothpaste.

5. **Brush all surfaces of the teeth, tongue, and gums.**
6. Hold emesis basin near the patient's chin and have the patient rinse their mouth. If they are unconscious or unable to rinse independently, use a swab to apply mouthwash to the gums, tongues, and mucous membranes in the mouth.
7. Floss the teeth (optional).
8. Wipe the mouth dry and remove the towel from the patient's chest.
9. Put used linens in the soiled linen hamper.
10. Rinse toothbrush and empty, rinse, and dry the basin.
11. Remove gloves and wash hands.
12. Report any bleeding or mouth sores to the nurse.

When providing oral care to an unconscious patient:
1. Turn the patient and the patient's head to the side so that excess fluid runs out of the mouth; this prevents the person from choking and aspiration.
2. Put on gloves.
3. Put a towel under the patient's face and a kidney basin under the chin.
4. Use a padded tongue blade to keep the patient's mouth open; never use force.
5. Using sponge swabs moistened with a cleaning agent, clean all surfaces of the teeth, gums, tongue, inside of cheek, and lips.
6. Remove supplies and wipe the patient's mouth.
7. Apply lubricant to the lips.

Skill: Cleaning Dentures

When brushing dentures, do NOT use a regular toothbrush, use a denture brush; regular toothbrushes can create scratches on the dentures, allowing bacteria to grow in it. Dentures should be cleaned as often as natural teeth. To brush dentures:
1. Put on gloves.
2. Line the sink with a washcloth to prevent denture breakage in case you drop the dentures. If you don't take any precautions to prevent denture breakage and the denture breaks, you may be charged with negligence.
3. Ask the patient to take off their dentures. If they need help:
   a. Have them open their mouth.
   b. Hold a gauze between your index and thumb, grasp the upper dentures and move it up and down slightly to break the seal. Remove the dentures and put it in the kidney basin.
   c. Hold a gauze between your index and thumb, grasp the lower dentures, turn them slightly and lift them out. Put the dentures in the kidney basin.
4. Holding the dentures over the sink, rinse the dentures before brushing. Use a denture brush, a toothette, or washcloth and tepid water to clean the dentures. Hot water can warp the dentures. Brush and rinse all surfaces of the dentures.
5. If dentures are to be stored:
   a. Put dentures in a denture cup with water and an effervescent denture tablet and return the covered denture cup to the patient's bedside table.

b. Use a toothbrush or swab to wash the patient's mouth. Rinse the mouth.

6. If dentures are to be reinserted:
   a. Use a toothbrush or swab to wash the patient's mouth. Rinse the mouth.
   b. Hold the upper dentures using your index and thumb, lift the patient's upper lip, and insert the dentures.
   c. Hold the lower dentures using your index and thumb, pull down the patient's lower lips, and insert the dentures.
7. Wipe the patient's mouth.
8. Report any bleeding or sores to the nurse.

Dressing and Grooming

Grooming involves dressing, hair care, shaving, nail care, and eyeglass and hearing aid care.

Dressing

Dress patients in their own clothing and encourage them to choose their clothing. Always check with them to see if they are dressed comfortably.

Skill: Undressing and Dressing a Patient

1. Adjust the bed to a comfortable working position. Lower the side rail nearest you.
2. Perform hand hygiene and put on gloves.
3. Cover the patient with a bath blanket. Pull top linens down to the foot of the bed.
4. Help the patient undress.
   a. If the garment fastens in the back:
      i. Lift the head and shoulders or turn the patient so that they are facing away from you.
      ii. Undo buttons, zippers, ties, etc.
      iii. Slide the garment from the shoulder down to the arm. If the patient is on their side, remove clothing from one side, turn the patient on their other side, and remove clothing. **Always remove clothing from the weak or paralyzed limb last.**
   b. If the garments fastens in the front:
      i. Undo buttons, zippers, ties, etc.
      ii. Slide the garment down from the shoulder to the arm, on the strongest side.
      iii. Lift the head and shoulders, bring the garment over to the weak side, and remove the garment.
      iv. If you cannot lift the patient's head and shoulders, turn the patient so they are lying on their weak side, tuck the removed half of garment under the patient. Turn the patient so that they are lying on their strong side, remove garment from the weak side.
   c. If removing a pullover garment:

    i.   Undo buttons, zippers, ties, etc.

    ii.   Remove the garment from the strong side.

    iii.   Lift the head and shoulders or turn the patient so they are lying on their weak side.

    iv.   Bring the garment up to the neck and then over the head.

    v.   Remove the garment from the patient's weak side.

d. If removing underwear or pants:

    i.   Remove footwear and socks.

    ii.   Undo buttons, zippers, ties, belts, etc.

    iii.   Ask the person to lift their buttocks. Slide underwear and pants down over hips and buttocks. Lower the buttocks.

    iv.   If the patient cannot lift their buttocks, turn the patient so that they are lying on their weak side. Slide underwear and pants, on the string side, off the hips and buttocks. Turn the patient so that they are lying on their strong side; slide underwear and pants, on the weak side, off the hips and buttocks.

    v.   Slide underwear and pants down the legs and feet.

5. Help the patient dress. **Always put garment on affected (weak) side first.**

a. Putting on garments that open in the back:

    i.   Slide garment onto arm and shoulder of the weak side.

    ii.   Slide garment onto arm and shoulder of the strong side.

    iii.   Lift the patient's head and shoulders. Button, zip, tie, etc. the back.

    iv.   If you cannot lift the patient's head and shoulders, turn the patient so they are lying on their strong side. Button, zip, tie, etc. the back.

b. Putting on garments that open in the front:

    i.   Slide garment onto arm and shoulder of the weak side.

    ii.   Lift the patient's head and shoulders. Bring garment around to the strong side and return the patient to the supine position. Guide the strong arm into the sleeve.

    iii.   If you cannot lift the patient's head and shoulders, turn the patient so that they are lying on their strong side. Place the garment so that it covers the back. Turn the patient so that they are lying on their weak side. Pull the garment out from underneath them. Position the patient so they are lying on their back. Guide the strong arm through the sleeve.

    iv.   Button, zip, tie, etc.

c. Putting on pullover garments:

    i.   Gather the top and bottom of the garment together at the neck opening.

    ii.   Pull the garment over the patient's head.

    iii.   Slide the weak arm through the sleeve.

    iv.   Slide the strong arm through the sleeve.

    v.   Lift the patient's head and shoulders and pull the garment down.

    vi.   If you cannot lift the patient's head and shoulders, turn the patient so they are lying on their strong side. Pull the garment down on the weak side.

Turn the patient so that they are lying on their weak side. Pull the garment down on the strong side.

    d. Putting on underwear or pants:
        i.   Slide underwear or pants over feet and up the legs.
        ii.   Ask the person to raise their hips and buttocks.
        iii. Bring underwear or pants up over the buttocks.
        iv. If the patient cannot raise their hips or buttocks:
            1. Turn the patient onto their strong side and pull underwear or pants, on the weak side, over the buttocks.
            2. Turn the patient onto their weak side and pull underwear or pants, on the strong side, over the buttocks.
        v.   Button, zip, tie, buckle, etc. pants.

6. Gather soiled garments and put them in the hamper.
7. Remove and dispose gloves. Practice hand hygiene.
8. Record and report any observations.

Changing A Gown On A Patient With An IV

1. Perform hand hygiene and put on gloves.
2. Place a bath blanket over the patient and pull top linens to the foot of the bed.
3. Turn the patient on their side so you can untie the gown.
4. Remove the gown from the arm with no IV.
5. On the arm with an IV, gather the sleeves and slide it over the IV site and tubing.
6. Remove the IV bag from the pole and slide the IV bag and tubing through the sleeve. Always keep the bag above the person.
7. Hang the IV bag on the pole.
8. Gather the sleeves (on the side of the IV site) of a clean gown, remove IV bag from the pole, and slide it through the sleeve. Re-hang the IV bag.
9. Slide the gathered sleeves over the IV tubing and onto the shoulder.
10. Slide opposite arm into opposite sleeve.
11. Tie the gown.
12. Pull top linens up and remove the the bath blanket.
13. Remove and discard gloves. Practice hand hygiene.
14. Report and record any observations.

Hair Care

Provide hair care as needed and before visitors arrive. Daily brushing increase blood flow to the scalp and helps keep hair soft and shiny by spreading oil from the scalp to the hair shaft. Use a wide-tooth comb for combing curly hair, as well as tangled hair.

Hair care may mean different things for different cultures, consult the patient and their family for how to care for their hair. Also, each facility may have different policies for hair care; in some facilities a doctor's order is needed for shampooing and in some facilities, hair care is handled by beauticians.

Record and report observations of the following:
- Scalp sores
- Flaking, itching, rash
- Patches of hair loss
- Very dry or oily hair
- Matted or tangled hair
- Signs of nits or lice
    - Nits are lice eggs; they are oval and yellow to white in color
    - Lice are the size of a sesame seed and grayish white in color

Depending on safety factors, a patient's hair may be shampooed during a shower or tub bath, shampooed at the sink, or shampooed in bed. Some facilities have shampoo caps that allow you to dry shampoo a patient's hair without needing to rinse the hair. Follow manufacturer instructions for using dry shampoo caps.

Shampooing Hair

1. Cover the person's chest with a bath towel.
2. Comb the hair to remove tangles.
3. Position the person.
    a. If shampooing at the sink, place a folded towel over the edge of the sink to protect the neck. The patient's head is tilted back over the sink with the neck placed on the sink edge. A water pitcher or hand-held nozzle is used to wet the hair.
    b. If shampooing in bed, position the patient so that their head and shoulders are at the edge of the bed. Place a waterproof pad and shampoo tray under the head to protect the bed from getting wet. Place towels under the neck for support if necessary.
4. If using a pitcher, fill the pitcher with water. Water temperature should be about 105F.
5. Have the patient hold a dry washcloth over the eye.
6. Practice proper hand hygiene and out on gloves.
7. Wet hair. Apply shampoo. Use both hands and wash the hair, starting at the hairline and working towards the back of the head. Use your fingertips to clean and massage the scalp, never use your fingernails.
8. Rinse the hair.
9. Apply conditioner and rinse.
10. Squeeze water out of the patient's hair and wrap the hair with a towel.
11. Remove the shampoo tray and waterproof pad.
12. Raise the head and dry the person's face.
13. Comb hair to remove tangles.
14. Dry and style hair.

15. Remove and discard gloves. Practice hand hygiene.
16. Record and report observations.

Shaving

Safety razors (blade razors) or electric razors are used to shave hair. Always use electric razors for patients using anticoagulant drugs or patient's with blood clotting issues. If using the facility's electric razor, clean it before and after use. Always shave hair in the correct direction:
- Shave in the direction of growth when shaving the face with safety razors.
- Shave in the direction of growth when shaving the underarms with safety razors.
- Shave against the direction of growth when shaving the legs with safety razors.
- Shave against the direction of growth when using electric shavers. Some states require that you shave in the direction of growth.

Shave legs and underarms after bathing; bathing softens the hair. Disposable safety razors should be disposed of in sharps containers.

Shaving the face:
1. Fill wash basin with warm water.
2. Place wash basin and shaving supplies on the over-bed table.
3. Help the patient to sit on the side of the bed or raise the head of the bed.
4. Place a towel over the patient's chest and shoulders.
5. Practice hand hygiene and put on gloves.
6. Wet a washcloth and apply to the patient's face for 2 to 3 minutes to soften the beard.
7. Apply shaving cream to the beard.
8. Hold the skin taut and shave in the direction of growth, rinsing the razor as needed.
9. Rinse off any remaining shaving cream and pat dry.
10. Apply after shave as requested. Do not apply after shave if there are any nicks or cuts.
11. Remove and discard gloves. Practice hand hygiene.
12. Record and report any observations.

Foot Care

Skill: Provide Foot Care On One Foot
1. Perform hand hygiene and put on gloves.
2. Fill basin with warm water. Check the temperature and ask patient to check the water.
3. Put basin on a protective barrier and in a comfortable position for the patient to put their foot in.
4. Put patient's foot in the water.
5. Apply soap to a wet washcloth.
6. Supporting the ankle and foot, lift foot from water and wash foot (including between the toes).
7. Rinse and dry foot and toes.
8. Apply lotion to the top and bottom of foot. Do NOT apply lotion between the toes.

9. Empty, rinse, and dry basin. Place basin in dirty supply area.
10. Put used linen/washcloth in soiled linen hamper.
11. Remove gloves and wash hands.

Nail Care

In most states, CNAs are not allowed to trim a patient's nails. If you notice a patient's nails needs trimming, notify a licensed nurse. Toenails can become thick with age or due to diabetes; patients with diabetes have poor circulation and poor wound healing so extra care must be taken with diabetic patients.

When washing a patient's hand, wash the underside of nails where dirt can accumulate. Soaking a patient's hands and feet in warm water can make nail trimming and cuticle care easier. Keep the area between fingers and toes dry (avoid lotion) to prevent bacterial growth and skin breakdown.

When cleaning the nails:
1. Soak nails in warm water for 10 to 20 minutes before cleaning.
2. Use an orangewood stick or wooden end of a cotton swab to clean under the nails.
3. Dry the hands and/or feet.
4. Use an emery board to file nail edges so that they are smooth.
5. Apply lotion; avoid getting lotion between fingers and/or toes.
6. Report and record any observations.

Fluids and Nutrition

Nutrition is the ingestion, digestion (breaking down of food into nutrients), absorption (transfer of nutrients from the digestive tract to the bloodstream), and metabolism (conversion of nutrients into energy) of food. There are 6 types of nutrients:
- Proteins: needed for tissue growth and repair; contains amino acids which are the "building blocks" of all body cells
- Carbohydrates: provide energy and fiber; source of glucose
- Fats: provide energy and help with absorbing fat-soluble vitamins
- Vitamins: can be fat-soluble (vitamins A,D,E, and K) or water-soluble (vitamin C and B-complex vitamins); needed for many body functions
- Minerals: needed for bone and tooth formation, nerve and muscle function, fluid balance, and other body processes
- Water: needed for all body processes

Nutrient	Source	Function
Vitamin A	Liver, leafy greens, egg yolk, carrots, milk	Vision, healthy mucous membranes/skin/hair, growth
Vitamin B1 (thiamin)	Pork, liver, breads, beans, peanuts	Energy, muscle tone, nerve function

Vitamin B2 (riboflavin)	Milk, leafy greens, liver, eggs	Protein and carbohydrate metabolism, eyes, healthy skin/mucous membranes
Vitamin B3 (niacin)	Meat, liver, fish, nuts	Protein, fat, and carbohydrate metabolism, digestive system function
Vitamin B12	Meat, eggs, milk, cheese	Forming red blood cells and hemoglobin
Folic acid	Green leafy vegetables, whole grains, poultry, fish	Forming red blood cells, protein metabolism
Vitamin C (ascorbic acid)	Citrus, tomatoes, strawberries	Tissue healing, iron absorption
Vitamin D	Sunlight, fish liver oils	Helps with calcium and phosphorus absorption for healthy bones
Vitamin E	Vegetable oils, milk, eggs, leafy greens	Forming red blood cells, muscle function
Vitamin K	Liver, leafy greens, egg yolks, whole grains	Blood clotting
Calcium	Milk, cheese, whole grains, beans, leafy greens	Teeth and bone formation, muscle contraction, heart function, blood clotting
Phosphorus	Meat, fish, poultry, beans, yolk, nuts	Teeth and bone formation; carbohydrate, protein, and fat metabolism
Iron	Liver, leafy greens, meat, eggs, whole grains	Used to produce hemoglobin (molecule that carries oxygen)
Iodine	Table salt and seafood	Thyroid gland function
Sodium	Table salt, most foods	Fluid balance, nerve function, heart and skeletal muscle contraction
Potassium	Whole grains, fruits, vegetables, beans, meat	Nerve function, muscle contraction, heart function

Nutritional needs vary based on a person's age, activity level, and health; it may also be affected by a person's ability to chew, difficulty swallowing (dysphagia), cultural considerations (religious restrictions, etc.), and emotional well-being (depression, etc.). Infants, young children, and teenagers need more calories and iron because they are growing. Pregnant and nursing women need more protein and calcium.

As people age, their sense of taste, smell, and thirst changes which can lead to nutrition and dehydration issues. Fluid can be lost through respiration, perspiration, evaporation, and elimination. Proper nutrition and hydration is needed for the body to function. Adequate hydration is needed to regulate body temperature and keep cellular functions operating properly.

Nutritional imbalances (too much salt, etc.), certain medications, and certain diseases can cause fluid to accumulate in the body; this is called edema. Signs of edema include swollen ankles, puffy eyes, abdominal swelling, and imprints on the skin from rings, socks, clothing that has become too tight. Edema can decrease the blood flow to an area, causing pain and possible damage to the body part. Notify the nurses if a patient has edema.

Patients may be placed on special diet plans for their nutritional needs; follow the patient's diet plan. If a patient refuses to eat according to their diet plan, it is considered non-compliance. Non-compliance can lead to malnutrition.

Diet Plan	Explanation
Regular diet	There are no restrictions; a well-balanced diet. May be tailored to increase or reduce calories for weight gain/loss. May be tailored to increase or reduce fiber for digestive issues. May be tailored to be more bland to reduce digestive tract irritation.
Mechanical diet	Foods that are hard to chew or digest are removed from the diet. A mechanical chopped diet is when food has been chopped to be easier to chew. A mechanical soft diet is when food has been pureed.
Pureed diet (mechanical soft diet)	Food is pureed and must be of thing consistency before serving it to the patient.
Carbohydrate controlled diet	Carbohydrate limited diet for diabetic patients. A dietician determines the amount of carbohydrates a patient should consume.
Clear liquid diet	A clear liquid diet is used when preparing patients for some medical procedures, when patients are recovering from a medical procedure, or when a patient is vomiting or nauseous. Foods that are considered clear liquids include water, gelatin, fat-free broth, clear juices, clear carbonated sodas, and coffee and tea (without cream).
Full liquid diet	A clear liquid diet plus any food that can be poured at room or body temperature (milk, frozen desserts, egg custards, cereal gruels, etc.)
Sodium restricted diet	Typically used for patients with hypertension, heart disease, or kidney disease. The patient may be allowed to have a small amount of salt or not salt at all.
Low cholesterol diet	Diet contains food with lower fat. Typically used for patients with heart disease.

Meal guidelines:

- Before serving a patient, check that the name of the meal tray matches the name of the patient.
- When referencing food on a plate, use a clock face as reference. For example, the potatoes are located at 3 o'clock.
- When feeding a patient, use a spoon instead of a fork.
- Give patients meal options, unless restricted by diet.
- Converse with patients and encourage social interactions.
- Keep hot food hot and cold food cold.
- Be patient with slow eaters.

Skill: Feeding Patients That Cannot Feed Themselves

1. Before feeding the patient, check the name of the meal tray and ask the client to state their name.
2. **Ensure the client is in a sitting position (75 to 90 degrees).**
3. Place the tray in front of the patient.
4. Clean the patient's hand.
5. Sit in a chair, facing the patient.
6. Tell the patient what foods and drinks are on the tray and ask them what they would like to eat first.
7. Offer one bite of each type of food, telling the patient what is in each bite.
8. Offer beverages to the patient throughout the meal.
9. Before offering the next bite or sip, ask the patient if they are ready for the next bite/sip.
10. At the end of the meal, clean the patient's hands and mouth.
11. Remove food tray.
12. Leave patient in a sitting position (75 to 90 degrees).
13. Wash hands.

Alternate Methods of Providing Nutrition

For patients that are unable to drink or eat, fluids and nutrition may be given through IV therapy, enteral nutrition, and/or total parenteral nutrition. Nurses manage IV therapy, enteral nutrition, and total parenteral nutrition; nursing assistants may help the nurse.

Intravenous (IV) therapy is a procedure that delivers fluids directly into a vein; nursing assistants do not manage IV therapy but may care for patients on IV therapy. IV therapy is not a complete source of nutrition, it only provides glucose, vitamins, and minerals.

Enteral nutrition (tube feeding) is a procedure where food, in liquid form, is delivered into the digestive tract; it is typically used for patients that cannot chew or swallow. For short term tube feeding (less than 6 weeks), a nasogastric or nasointestinal tube is used. For long term tube feeding, a gastrostomy, jejunostomy, or PEG tube. Feedings may be given at scheduled times or continuously through an infusion pump. Since patients receiving enteral nutrition therapy are at a higher risk for regurgitation and aspiration, the head of the patient's bed is raised during feedings and for at least 1 hour afterwards. Avoid left side-lying positions which can prevent the stomach from emptying into the small intestine.

- Nasogastric tube: tube is inserted through nose and into the stomach
- Nasointestinal tube: tube is inserted through nose and into the small intestine
- Gastrostomy tube: tube is inserted into the stomach through an abdominal surgical incision
- Jejunostomy tube: tube is inserted into the jejunum through an abdominal surgical incision
- Percutaneous endoscopic gastrostomy (PEG): a gastrostomy tube that is inserted into the stomach through the mouth and throat instead of through an abdominal surgical incision

Signs that a patient may have regurgitated or aspirated a feeding:

- Nausea, bloating, or pain during a feeding
- Coughing, gagging, or vomiting during a feeding
- Abdominal distention

Patients that may not be able to tolerate food in the digestive tract (very ill, recovering from gastrointestinal surgery, etc.) may need total parenteral nutrition (TPN) therapy. TPN therapy is able to provide complete nutrition needs. In TPN therapy, nutrition is delivered directly into the bloodstream through a catheter inserted into a large vein near the heart. Patients on TPN therapy are at increased risk for infections, fluid imbalances, and blood sugar imbalances. Notify the nurse if you observe the following:

- Fevers, chills
- Chest pain
- Difficulty breathing
- Nausea, vomiting, diarrhea
- Thirst
- Sweating
- Trembling
- Confusion or behavioral changes
- Signs/symptoms of diabetes

Patients with feeding tubes are not allowed to eat or drink; provide oral hygiene, lubricate lips, and rinse the mouth every 2 hours for patient comfort. For patients with nasogastric or nasointestinal tubes, clean the nose and nostrils every 4 to 8 hours. Secure the tube to the nose and shoulder area to prevent pulling and dangling of the tube.

Fluid Balance

Adults need 1500 mL of water daily to survive; adults need 2000 to 2500 mL of water for normal fluid balance. Infants and young children are more sensitive to fluid loss. Older adults have decreased thirst sensation so should be reminded more often to drink water.

Recording Intake and Output

Liquids should be measured in cubic centimeters (cc) or milliliters (mL). 1 fluid ounce is equal to 30 mL. Foods that are liquid at room or body temperature (ice cream, gelatin, pudding, etc.) are considered liquids. Fluid intake also includes IV fluids and enteral or TPN feedings, though the nurse, not the nursing assistant, will be responsible for recording these amounts. Fluid output includes urine, vomit, blood, wound drainage, and diarrhea.

Measuring fluid intake:

1. Record the amount of liquid ingested by a patient; this includes foods that are considered to be liquid. You should be familiar with the amount of fluid in commonly served items.
2. If a patient doesn't finish the entire serving of an item, pour the remaining liquid into a graduate and calculate the intake by subtracting the amount in the graduate from the amount contained in the full serving.

Measuring fluid output:

1. Before flushing the urine down the toilet, pour the urine into a graduated cylinder. Place the graduate on a flat surface and read the urine amount at eye level.
2. Clean and disinfect the graduate and urine receptacle and remove gloves.
3. Record your observations (color, amount, odor, clarity, etc.)

Skill: Measure and Record Urinary Output
1. Put on gloves before handling bedpan.
2. Bring the bedpan to the toilet and pour the contents of the bedpan into the measuring container.
3. Rinse the bedpan and pour the rinse into the toilet.
4. Measure the urine at eye level with the container on a flat surface. If the urine is between measurement lines, round up to the nearest 25 ml/cc.
5. Empty the contents of the measuring container into the toilet.
6. Rinse the measuring container and pour the rinse into the toilet.
7. Remove gloves and wash hands.
8. Record output.

Elimination

The average adult produces 800 to 2000 mL of urine a day. Infants produce 200 to 300 mL of urine a day. Notify a nurse if an infant does not have a wet diaper for several hours.

Normal stool is brown. Black or tarry stools may indicate bleeding in the stomach or small intestines. Bright red stools may indicate bleeding in the lower colon or rectum. Food may also affect the color of stool. Breast fed infants have yellow stools that are very soft. Formula fed infants have yellowish-brown or greenish-brown stools.

With age, the need to urinate or defecate decreases. Decreased appetite and thirst, medication, inactivity, weak pelvic muscles and slower digestion increase the risk for constipation. Prolonged constipation can lead to fecal impaction (when stool is stuck in the colon and can't be pushed out). Signs and symptoms of fecal impaction include cramps, bloating, and stool leakage. Diarrhea occurs when waste passes too quickly, not allowing the body to absorb the water. It can cause anal skin irritation, dehydration, and electrolyte imbalances. Notify licensed nurses when patients are suffering from constipation or diarrhea to prevent further complications.

Guidelines:
- Normal urine is clear and pale yellow, straw-colored, or amber. Report any abnormalities in urine color, clarity, and odor.
- Help patients with elimination needs on a routine basis to establish a pattern and avoid accidents.
- Perform proper skin care after elimination.
- Help patients wash their hands after elimination.
- Observe, report, and record excess or decreased output.

Urinary Elimination Problems
- Dysuria: pain or difficulty urinating.
- Hematuria: blood in urine.
- Nocturia: frequent urination at night.
- Oliguria: less than 500 mL of urine in 24 hours.
- Polyuria: large volumes of urine.
- Urinary incontinence: involuntary leakage of urine.
- Urinary retention: inability to urinate.
- Urinary urgency: sudden and urgent need to urinate.

Skill: Helping A Patient Use A Bedpan
1. Practice hand hygiene and put on gloves.
2. Adjust the bed to a comfortable working height. Lower the head of the bed so that the bed is a flat as possible or as much as tolerated by the patient.
3. Fan fold top linens down far enough to place the bedpan.

4. Place a protective pad under the patient's buttocks.
5. Adjust gown or garment to expose the buttocks.
6. Have the patient turn or roll so that they are facing away from you and place the bedpan under the patient. A fracture pan might be needed for immobilized patients. Turn/roll them back so they are in the supine position.
7. Remove and discard gloves. Practice hand hygiene.
8. Raise the head of the bed so that the patient is in a sitting position.
9. Give the patient some tissues before leaving the room.
10. When the patient signals that they are done, enter the room. Knock before entering.
11. Practice hand hygiene and put on gloves.
12. Fan fold top linens to the foot of the bed.
13. Lower the head of the bed and ask the patient to raise their buttocks or roll the patient away from the bedpan.
14. Clean the genital area if the patient cannot do so themselves.
15. Remove and discard the protective pad.
16. Remove the bedpan and empty contents into a toilet. Remove one of your gloves if you need to raise the side rails or touch a doorknob.
17. Rinse and disinfect the bedpan. Place bedpan in designated dirty supply area.
18. Remove and dispose of gloves. Practice hand hygiene and put on clean gloves.
19. Help the patient wash their hands.
20. Remove and discard gloves. Practice hand hygiene.
21. Report and record your observations.

Helping A Patient Use A Urinal

1. Depending on the patient's preference, the patient may use the urinal while lying, sitting, or standing.
2. Perform hand hygiene and put on gloves.
3. Hand the patient the urinal.
4. Give the patient some tissues before leaving the room.
5. Remove and discard gloves. Practice hand hygiene
6. When the patient signals that they are done, enter the room. Knock before entering.
7. Practice hand hygiene and put on gloves.
8. Clean the genital area if the patient cannot do so themselves.
9. Remove and discard gloves. Practice hand hygiene and put on new gloves.
10. Take the urinal to the bathroom. Empty the urinal into the toilet (do not empty the urinal if anything unusual should be observed by the nurse).
11. Clean and disinfect the urinal. Return the urinal to the proper place.
12. Help the patient wash their hands.
13. Remove and discard gloves. Practice hand hygiene.
14. Record and report any observations.

Catheter Care

Common catheters types include straight catheters and indwelling catheters. Straight catheters are used to empty the bladder and are then removed. Indwelling catheters (retention or Foley catheters) remain in the bladder, allowing for urine to constantly drain. There are two types of urine drainage bags: standard drainage bags and leg bags. Standard drainage bags hold at least 2000 mL of urine. Leg bags hold less than 1000 mL of urine and are attached to the thigh or calf. Standard drainage bags are used when a person is in bed.

Catheter tubes and drainage should be kept free of kinks and below the bladder to allow urine to flow freely. Catheters should be secured to the upper thigh to prevent tugging and friction at the insertion site.

Catheters increase the risk for urinary tract infections (UTIs) so it is important to provide proper catheter care.

Skill: Provide Catheter Care

1. Practice hand hygiene and put on gloves.
2. Provide patient privacy and adjust the bed to a comfortable height. Lock the wheels.
3. Fill a wash basin with warm water (110F to 115F) and place it, along with soap, towels, and washcloths, next to the bed.
4. Cover the patient with a bath blanket and fan fold top linens to the foot of the bed.
5. Place waterproof pad under the patient's buttocks.
6. Expose the perineal area.
7. Ask the patient to spread their legs and bend their knees.
8. Check the drainage tubing for any kinks.
9. Provide perineal care.
10. Wet another clean washcloth and apply soap.
11. **Hold the catheter at the meatus (near urethra opening) and continue to hold it there throughout the procedure to prevent tugging the catheter.**
12. **Clean the catheter from the meatus down the catheter at least 4 inches. Use circular and downward strokes, moving away from the meatus. Use a clean area of the washcloth for each stroke.**
13. **Use a new washcloth and the same method as washing the catheter to rinse the catheter.**
14. Use a new washcloth to dry the catheter and perineal area.
15. Secure the tubing to the upper thigh and remove the waterproof pad.
16. Remove and discard gloves. Practice hand hygiene and put on gloves.
17. Pull top linens up and remove the bath blanket.
18. Remove and discard gloves. Practice hand hygiene.
19. Report and record observations.

Emptying a Urine Drainage Bag

1. Practice hand hygiene and put on gloves.
2. Put paper towels on the floor and then put the graduate on top of it.
3. Open the clamp at the bottom of the drainage bag and let urine flow into the graduate. Be careful to not let the drain touch the graduate.
4. Clean the end of the drain with alcohol and close it.
5. Measure the urine output and record your observations.
6. Empty the graduate into the toilet. If there is anything a nurse should see, do not empty the graduate until the nurse has seen it.
7. Clean equipment and return it to the storage area.
8. Remove and discard gloves. Practice hand hygiene.

Removing Indwelling Catheters

Indwelling catheters have two lumens and a balloon. To inflate the balloon, sterile water is injected, using a syringe, through 1 lumen. Urine drains through the other lumen. To remove the catheter, you will need to deflate the balloon. You will use a syringe to draw water out of the balloon. The nurse will tell you what size syringe is needed.

1. Practice hand hygiene and put on gloves.
2. Cover the patient with a bath blanket and fan fold top linens to the foot of the bed.
3. Expose the perineal area.
4. Get the correct sized syringe. You must know how much water is in the balloon because you must draw out all the water from the balloon; otherwise you can injured the urethra when removing the catheter. If there are 10 mL of water in the balloon and you were only able to draw out 9 mL, do not remove the catheter and immediately notify the nurse.
5. Remove the tape or tube holder that is securing the catheter to the patient.
6. Place a towel between the legs, for a female, or over the thighs, for a male.
7. Remove water from the balloon.
    a. Pull the syringe plunger back to the 0.5 mL mark.
    b. Attach the syringe to the catheter's balloon port.
    c. Allow water to drain into the syringe. Do not pull back on the plunger; notify the nurse if the water is draining slowly or not at all. Be sure to drain all of the water from the balloon.
8. Once all the water has been drained from the balloon, pull the catheter gently and straight out.
9. Discard the catheter.
10. Dry the perineal area with a towel.
11. Discard soiled items.
12. Remove and discard gloves. Practice hand hygiene and put on clean gloves.
13. Bring top linens up and remove bath blanket.
14. Remove and discard gloves. Practice hand hygiene.

15. Record and report observations.

Applying a Condom Catheter

Condom catheters are changed daily after perineal care. The nurse will tell you what size to use. Do not apply a condom catheter if the penis is red or irritated.

1. Practice hand hygiene and put on gloves.
2. Provide patient privacy and adjust the bed to a comfortable height.
3. Follow process for covering a patient with a bath blanket and exposing the perineal area.
4. Place a waterproof pad under the patient's buttocks.
5. Remove the old condom catheter, if any.
   a. Remove tape and roll condom off the penis.
   b. Disconnect the drainage tube from the condom and cap the tube.
6. Provide perineal care.
7. Remove and discard gloves. Practice hand hygiene and put on new gloves.
8. Expose the condom's adhesive surface.
9. Roll the condom catheter onto the penis, leaving one inch of space between the penis tip and end of catheter.
10. Secure the condom.
    a. Self-adhering condoms: press condom to penis.
    b. Secure with tape: apply tape in a spiral; do not completely encircle the penis, it can block blood flow.
11. Connect the condom to drainage tubing.
12. Tape the catheter to the patient's inside thigh.
13. Secure the drainage bag to the bed frame; do not secure it to a movable part of the bed.
14. Remove waterproof pad.
15. Cover the person and remove the bath blanket.
16. Remove and discard gloves. Practice hand hygiene.
17. Record and report observations.

Administering a Cleansing Enema

A suppository is a small, round, or cone-shaped drug that is inserted into a body opening, where it dissolves. Because it is a drug, nursing assistants do not generally insert suppositories. An enema is an injection of fluid into the rectum or lower colon to relieve constipation, fecal impaction, etc. Cleansing enemas clear the bowel of feces and are typically given before certain surgical/medical procedures. Small volume enemas are given for constipation or when the bowel does not need to be completely cleared. Report any signs of enema retention such as abdominal distension or pain. Passing stools, gas, or watery brown fluid is expected.

1. Practice hand hygiene and put on gloves.
2. Prepare the enema solution in a bathroom.
   a. Close the clamp on the tube.

b. Fill the enema bag with lukewarm water. The nurse will tell you the temperature (typically, 105F) and amount of water to use.

c. Prepare the enema solution.

    i. Tap water enemas: add nothing.

    ii. Saline enemas: add salt as directed.

    iii. Soapsuds enemas: add castile soap as directed.

d. Stir or gently rotate the enema bag; do not shake. Scoop off any soap suds.

e. Release the clamp on the tubing and let a little water out; this is done to get air out of the bag.

f. Re-clamp the tubing.

3. Collect supplies, hang the enema bag on an IV pole, and place them near the bedside.

4. Cover the patient with a bath blanket. Fan-fold top linens to the foot of the bed.

5. Position the patient on their left side in Sim's position.

6. Adjust the IV pole so that the enema bag is 12 inches above the anus.

7. Place a waterproof pad under the buttocks.

8. Expose the buttocks.

9. Lubricate the top 2 to 4 inches of the enema tube.

10. Ask the patient to take a deep breath and exhale slowly as you insert the enema tube into the anus (directing tubing toward umbilicus and no more than 3 to 4 inches for an adult). If you encounter resistance, stop and call the nurse.

11. Unclamp the tubing and allow the solution to run. If the person complains of pain, nausea, etc., clamp the tube. Unclamp when symptoms subside. Stop if the patient cannot tolerate the procedure.

12. The tube should be clamped before the enema bag is empty to prevent air from entering the anus.

13. Remove tubing and ask the patient to hold the enema solution for as long as ordered.

14. Help the patient to the bathroom or have them use a bedpan.

15. Discard equipment and supplies.

16. Return to the room when the patient signals. Practice hand hygiene and put on gloves.

17. Observe the stool for amount, color, and consistency. Call the nurse to observe the results. Flush contents down the toilet after the nurse observes the results.

18. Provide perineal care, if needed.

19. Remove waterproof underpad.

20. Clean and disinfect equipment.

21. Remove and discard gloves. Practice hand hygiene and put on new gloves.

22. Help the patient wash their hands.

23. Remove and discard gloves. Practice hand hygiene.

24. Record and report observations.

Changing an Ostomy Pouch

Stools irritate the skin, so it's important to keep the skin washed and dried; a skin barrier should also be applied around the stoma. Ostomy pouches have a drain at the bottom that can be opened to empty the pouch; the drain can also be open when the pouch balloons, to release flatus. Wipe the drain with toilet paper before closing.

Frequent pouch changes can irritate the skin, so pouches are only changed every 2 to 7 days and when there is a leak. Keep the area dry for 1 to 2 hours after a change to allow the adhesive time to seal with the skin.

Tight clothing should be avoided because it can prevent stool from entering the pouch.

1. Practice hand hygiene and put on gloves.
2. Cover the patient with a bath blanket and fan fold top linens to the foot of the bed.
3. Place a waterproof pad under the buttocks.
4. Remove the ostomy bag and skin barrier and dispose of them according to agency policy.
5. Wipe, cleanse, and dry the stoma and skin around it.
6. If ordered, apply skin protectant or barrier around the stoma.
7. If an ostomy belt is used, put a clean ostomy belt on the patient.
8. Remove the adhesive backing on the new ostomy pouch.
9. Pull the skin around the stoma taut; the skin must be wrinkle free.
10. Center the ostomy pouch over the stoma, making sure that the drain is pointed down.
11. Press around the edges to seal the ostomy pouch to the skin.
12. Connect the ostomy pouch to the ostomy belt, if an ostomy belt is used.
13. Remove the waterproof underpad.
14. Remove and discard gloves. Practice hand hygiene.
15. Report and record any observations.

Exercise and Activity

Bedrest

There are 3 types of bedrest. The patient's care plan and your assignment sheet will tell you what activities are allowed for the patient. Always ask the nurse what bedrest means for each patient.

- Strict bedrest: everything is done for the patient; the patient is in bed for all activities of daily living
- Bedrest: self-feeding, oral hygiene, bathing, shaving, and hair care are allowed
- Bedrest with commode privileges: commode is used for elimination
- Bedrest with bathroom privileges: the patient may leave the bed to use the bathroom for elimination

Complications from bedrest include:
- Pressure ulcers
- Constipation
- Blood clots
- Contracture
  - Abnormal shortening/hardening of muscles that leads to deformity and rigidity of joints
  - Common site for contractures are fingers, wrists, elbows, toes, knees, ankles, hips, neck, and spine
- Atrophy
  - Wasting of muscle tissue
- Orthostatic hypotension (postural hypotension)
  - Abnormally low blood pressure when standing up suddenly
  - Patient may feel weak and/or faint

Supportive devices may be used to position patients to prevent complications.
- Place the soles of feet flush against the footboard to prevent plantar flexion and foot-drop (permanent plantar flexion).
- Trochanter roll prevent hips and legs from turning out.
- Hip abduction wedges are used to keep hips apart.
- Use foam rubber sponges, rubber balls, hand rolls or grips to prevent contractures of the wrist and fingers.
- Bed cradles keep the weight of top linens off the feet to prevent foot-drop and pressure ulcers.

Exercise

Being able to move, walk, or exercise not only improves patients' circulation and musculoskeletal functioning, it helps patients feel more independent.

Range of Motion Exercises

Range of motion exercises are typically done at least twice a day or as ordered by the doctor. Do not push a joint past a point where pain occurs. Follow facility policies for exercising the neck.

Range of motion includes:
- Abduction: moving the limb away from the body's midline
- Adduction: moving the limb toward the body's midline
- Flexion: bending the limb
- Extension: the opposite of flexion; a straightening movement that increases the angle between body parts.
- Dorsiflexion: bending foot up at the ankle
- Plantar flexion: bending foot down at the ankle
- Internal rotation: turning a joint inward
- External rotation: turning a joint outward
- Pronation: turning a joint downward
- Supination: turning a joint upward

Performing passive range of motion exercises:
1. Perform hand hygiene and put on gloves.
2. Adjust the bed to a comfortable height and lock the wheels.
3. Have the patient lie on their back.
4. Check the care plan to see how many repetitions to perform per exercise.
5. Exercise the shoulder.
    a. Raise the straight arm over the head and then lower it.
    b. Move the straight arm away from the side of the body to shoulder level and then return towards the body.
    c. Bend the elbow and raise the elbow to shoulder level. Lower and raise the forearm.
6. Exercise the elbow.
    a. Hold the patient's wrist and bend the elbow so that the fingers touch the shoulder.
    b. Straighten the arm.
7. Exercise the forearm.
    a. Turn the hand so that the palm is faced up and then turn it so the palm is faced down.
8. Exercise the wrist.
    a. Flex, extend, and rotate each wrist.
9. Exercise the thumb.
    a. Abduct, adduct, flex, and extend the thumb. Touch each fingertip with the thumb.
10. Exercise the fingers.
    a. Spread the fingers and thumbs apart and then bring them together.
    b. Make a fist with the thumb and fingers.

      c. Straighten the fingers.

11. Exercise the hips.
    a. Straighten and raise the leg. Lower the leg.
    b. Abduct, adduct, and rotate the leg.

12. Exercise the knees.
    a. Bend and straighten the knees.

13. Exercise the ankle.
    a. Turn the foot upward at the ankle.
    b. Turn the foot downward (toes pointing down).

14. Exercise the toes.
    a. Spread the toes and then bring them together.
    b. Curl and straighten the toes.

Skill: Perform Passive Range of Motion For One Knee and One Ankle

1. Perform hand hygiene and put on gloves.
2. Have the patient lie on their back and tell them to tell you if they are in pain.
3. Adjust the bed to a comfortable working height and lock the wheels.
4. **Support the leg at the knees and ankles. Bend and straighten the knees at least 3 times (stop if the patient complains of pain).**
5. **Support the foot and ankle. Turn the foot upward and downward (toes pointing down) at least 3 times (stop if the patient complains of pain).**
6. Lower the bed.
7. Wash hands.

Skill: Perform Passive Range of Motion For One Shoulder

1. Perform hand hygiene and put on gloves.
2. Have the patient lie on their back and tell them to tell you if they are in pain.
3. Adjust the bed to a comfortable working height and lock the wheels.
4. **Support the arm at the elbow and wrist. Raise the patient's straight arm over the head and then lower it. Do this at least 3 times, stop if the patient complains of pain.**
5. **Support the arm at the elbow and wrist. Move the patient's straight arm away from the side of the body to shoulder level and then return towards the body. Do this at least 3 times, stop if the patient complains of pain.**
6. Lower the bed.
7. Wash hands.

Canes and Walkers

Canes and walkers are used to help patients walk. Canes should be held 6 to 10 inches to the side and 6 to 10 inches in front of the strong foot. Walkers should be held 6 to 8 inches in front of the feet.

Rest/Sleep/Comfort

Adequate rest is essential to well-being and health. Pain and discomfort can interfere with rest and sleep. Signs a patient is possibly in pain (even if they deny it) include:

- changes in vital signs: rapid heart rate (tachycardia), increased respiration (tachypnea), difficulty breathing (dyspnea), high blood pressure (hypertension)
- loss of appetite, insomnia (inability to sleep)
- withdrawing from social and recreational activities
- sweating, crying, grunting, moaning, grimacing, etc.

There are 4 major types of pain:

- Acute pain: sudden pain from injury, trauma, disease, or surgery
- Chronic pain: persistent pain that lasts from months to years
- Radiating pain: pain that is felt at the site of injury as well as nearby areas
- Phantom pain: pain felt in a body part that is no longer there

If a patient complains of pain, obtain the following information and report it to the nurse:

- Location of pain
- Onset and duration
- Intensity of pain
- Factors that cause the pain (i.e. is there anything the patient does that brings on the pain?)
- Factors that affect the pain (i.e. is there anything the patient does that makes the pain better or worse?)
- Ask the patient to describe the pain
- Take their vital signs
- Ask the patient if they have other signs and symptoms (e.g., nausea, weakness, tingling, etc.)

Licensed nurses may give patients analgesics or pain medication. It is the CNA's responsibility to observe the patient's reaction to the medication, including changes to vital signs after taking the medication, effectiveness of pain relief, adverse reactions (also known as adverse drug effect), etc. and report them. Sudden drops in blood pressure or respirations, body rashes, and signs of distress need to be reported to the licensed nurse immediately.

Too much sleeping during the day can interfere with sleeping at night; it may also be a sign of an illness. Report any changes in consciousness or alertness to a licensed nurse promptly.

Sleep guidelines:

- Establish a routine to help patients sleep.
- Use positioning devices to increase comfort.
- Keep the bed in the lowest position.

- Lock wheelchairs when residents are sitting.
- Keep urinals, bedpans, or bedside commodes near the bed.
- Keep a night light on for when patients need to use the restroom at night.
- Avoid caffeinated products at least 3 to 4 hours before bedtime.

Musculoskeletal Injuries

Heat and cold applications are often used to treat musculoskeletal injuries or issues such as sprains and arthritis. Moist heat applications (water is in contact with the skin) penetrate deeper and faster than dry heat applications, so lower temperatures are used. Dry heat applications don't penetrate as deep, but the heat lasts longer. Moist cold applications also penetrate deeper and faster than dry cold applications, so higher temperatures are used. Be especially careful with applying heat or cold applications to older patients, patients with fair skin, and patients with decreased sensation. Heat and cold applications are applied no longer than 15 to 20 minutes and the skin is observed every 5 minutes.

Heat Applications

Heat relieves pain, relaxes muscles, decreases joint stiffness, and increases blood flow by dilating the vessels. However, if heat is applied too long, it can burn the skin as well as constrict blood vessels. Do not apply heat to areas that may have implants because metal conducts heat. Also, never apply heat to a pregnant woman's stomach; heat can affect the fetus.

Examples of moist heat applications:
- Hot compress
- Hot soak
- Sitz bath: perineal and rectal areas are immersed in warm or hot water
- Hot pack: a body part is wrapped with a dry or wet heat application

Cold Applications

Cold applications reduce pain and swelling, decreases circulation and bleeding by constricting blood vessels, and cools fevers. When a cold application is applied too long, patients can be at risk for burns and blisters and poor circulation. Cold compresses are examples of moist cold applications. Ice bags, ice collars, and ice gloves are examples of dry cold applications.

Applying Heat or Cold Applications

1. Practice hand hygiene and put on gloves.
2. Position the patient and expose the area to be treated.
3. For a hot or cold compress:
   a. For a hot compress, fill a basin with hot water.
   b. For a cold compress, place a small basin with cold water into a large basin with ice.
   c. Measure the temperature.
   d. Place the compress in the water, wring it out, and apply it to the area to be treated. Note the time.
   e. Cover the compress with a plastic wrap and towel or apply an aquathermia pad.

4. For a hot soak:
    a. Fill a basin with hot water and measure the temperature.
    b. Place the body part in the water and note the time.
    c. If necessary, cover the person with a bath blanket for warmth.
5. For a sitz bath:
    a. Put the disposable sitz bath on the toilet seat.
    b. Fill the sitz bath ⅔ full of water and measure the temperature.
    c. Secure the patient's gown above the waist.
    d. Have the patient sit on the sitz bath and note the time.
    e. If necessary, cover the person with a bath blanket for warmth.
6. For an aquathermia pad:
    a. Fill the heating unit to the fill line with distilled water (tap water contains minerals that can corrode the unit).
    b. Place the pad and tubing at the same level as the heating unit.
    c. Set the temperature as directed by a nurse (typically, 105F) and remove the key.
    d. Place the pad in the cover.
    e. Plug in the unit and let the water reach the desired temperature.
    f. Apply the pad to the area to be treated. Note the time.
    g. Secure the pad.
7. For a hot or cold pack:
    a. Follow manufacturer instructions for preparing the pack.
    b. Pace the pack in the cover and apply it to the area to be treated. Note the time.
    c. Secure the pack.
8. For an ice bag, collar, or glove:
    a. Check for leaks by filling the ice bag, collar, or glove with water and then empty the device.
    b. Fill the device with crushed ice or ice chips.
    c. Remove excess air from the device and then close the device.
    d. Dry the outside of the device and put the device in the cover.
    e. Apply the device to the area to be treated. Note the time.
    f. Secure the device.
9. Check the patient for signs of complications every 5 minutes. Hot and cold applications are applied for no longer than 15 to 20 minutes.

Cast Care

- Do not cover casts with blankets or other materials. As casts dry, they give off heat and can burn patients if the heat isn't allowed to escape.
- Turn the patient every 2 hours or as directed to dry the cast.
- Do not place a wet cast on a hard surface or put pressure on a wet cast, it can misshapen the cast.
- Casted arms or legs should be elevated to prevent swelling.

- Tell patients to not insert anything into the cast to scratch themselves; scratches can lead to infections.
- All jewelry should be removed from fingers and toes.
- Report signs and symptoms of the following:
    - Pain which can indicate ulcers, poor circulation, nerve damage
    - Signs of infections such as odor, fever, nausea, vomiting, drainage
    - Signs of reduced blood flow such as swelling, tightness, pale or blue skin
    - Temperature changes
    - Inability to move toes or fingers
    - Numbness

Musculoskeletal Disorders

Arthritis

There are two types of arthritis:
- Osteoarthritis: occurs when the cartilage on the end of bones is worn down; typically affects the hands, knees, hips, and spine
- Rheumatoid Arthritis: an autoimmune disease that attacks the lining of the joints; typically affects the wrist and fingers, but can affect the joints of the entire body.

There is no cure for arthritis. Arthritis is treated with pain and anti-inflammation drugs; heat and cold applications; exercise; weight control; etc.

Fractures

A fracture is a broken bone. There are many types of fractures:
- Simple fracture: the bone is broken in 1 place
- Closed fracture: the bone is broken, but the skin is intact
- Open (Compound) fracture: the bone and skin is broken
- Greenstick fracture: bone is bent and splintered, but not broken
- Impacted fracture: broken end of bones are pushed into each other
- Comminuted fracture: bone is broken into many little pieces

Signs and symptoms of fractures include:
- Pain and swelling
- Loss of function or movement
- Deformity
- Movement where movement should not occur
- Bruising
- Bleeding

Fractures are treated using the following procedures:
- Reduction: broken ends of bones are brought into alignment through manual manipulation or surgery
- Fixation: bone is held in place until the fracture heals
  - External fixation: bone is held in place without surgery using casts, splints, etc.
  - Internal fixation: bone is held in place using pins, screws, rods, etc. placed during surgery
- Traction: bones are put into alignment and traction unit is applied to exert a constant pull to keep the bones in alignment; traction is used until the fracture can be permanently repaired through surgery or casting

People over 65 years old, people that have osteoporosis, and people on drugs that weaken their bones or cause dizziness are at higher risk for falls and hip fractures. When treating patients with hip fractures:

- Prevent external rotation of the hip
- Keep the hip abducted and do not exercise the affected leg
- Do not let the person put weight on the affected leg unless ordered by a doctor
- Tell patients to not cross their legs
- Introduce weight bearing exercises to strengthen bones when appropriate as ordered by the care plan

Osteoporosis

Osteoporosis is a disease that causes bones to become weak and brittle. It typically affects older people, especially women who have gone through menopause. Patients who have osteoporosis are at high risk for fractures; even mild activity can cause fractures.

Loss of Limb

Amputation is the removal of a limb. Gangrene is tissue death caused by lack of blood supply; if gangrene isn't treated, it can spread and cause death. Gangrene often requires the tissue to be amputated. Patients who have had limbs amputated may experience phantom pain, among other issues such as anger, depression, etc. Phantom pain is pain that feels like it comes from a body part that is no longer there. Phantom pain can occur for a short period or for years after an amputation.

Respiratory Disorders

Respiratory disorders can be acute or chronic. Examples of acute respiratory problems include choking, allergic reaction, etc. Examples of chronic respiratory problems include chronic obstructive lung disease (COPD), emphysema, asthma, etc. Both acute and chronic respiratory problems can lead to hypoxia (lack of oxygen to body tissues) if not treated properly and promptly; hypoxia can lead to organ damage, brain damage, and/or death. When assessing a patient's breathing, consider the rate, depth, and ease of breathing as well as skin color and alertness.

Patients in respiratory distress may have the following signs and symptoms:
- Dyspnea: shortness of breath
- Cyanosis: bluish skin color
- Hypotension: low blood pressure
- Tachycardia: rapid heart rate
- Apnea: respiratory arrest (not breathing)
- Hypoventilation: breathing is slow and shallow, may also be irregular
- Hyperventilation: breathing is rapid and deeper than normal
- Kussmaul respirations: very deep and rapid breathing, may signal a diabetic coma
- Cheyne-Stokes respirations: abnormal pattern of breathing characterized by alternating cycles of deep breathing, shallow and slow breathing, and apnea; common when death is near
- Act confused and combative

If a patient goes into respiratory and/or cardiac arrest, begin CPR.

Influenza (Flu)

Influenza is a viral respiratory infection. The CDC recommends all persons 6 months or older should get the flu vaccine unless the person has a life-threatening allergy to the the vaccine. Signs and symptoms include fever, headache, aches and pain, weakness, cough, sore throat, etc.

Pneumonia

Pneumonia is a lung infection that causes the alveoli (air sacs) to fill up with fluid. Pneumonia can be a complication of the flu. Signs and symptoms include fever, coughing, chest pain when breathing, rapid pulse, shortness of breath, tiredness, muscle aches, etc.

Tuberculosis (TB)

Tuberculosis is a bacterial infection of the lungs that is highly contagious; it spreads through airborne droplets. Latent TB is when a person is infected with TB, but doesn't have any symptoms. A person is only contagious when they have an active TB infection. Patients with TB can be treated in long term care facilities only if there are environmental controls in place and the facility has a respiratory protection program. Wear a TB respirator when treating a TB patient or entering the home or room of a TB patient. TB patients should wear masks when being transported, in waiting areas, and when others are present.

Signs and symptoms of TB include coughing, sputum that may contain blood, weight loss, loss of appetite, fatigue, fever, night sweats, etc.

Oxygen Therapy

The doctor may order oxygen therapy for a patient. You may not administer oxygen; only licensed nurses can administer oxygen. However, do check or confirm with the care plan to see that the flow rate is correct; notify the nurse immediately if the flow rates do not match.

Oxygen therapy can be very drying to a patient's mucous membranes so moisture is often added to supplemental oxygen using a humidifier bottle. Check the humidifier bottle water level often and also check that there are bubbles in the bottle (which indicates that oxygen is flowing through the bottle).

Below is a list of oxygen sources:
- Oxygen tank: small tank that is sued for emergencies and transfers; also used by patients who walk or use wheelchairs. The nurse sets the flow meter rate. There is a gage that indicates the amount of oxygen remaining in the tank; notify the nurses when oxygen levels are low or the flow rate is incorrect.
- Oxygen concentrator: takes in oxygen from the air and delivers it to the patient.
- Liquid oxygen tank: small, lightweight, and portable unit containing liquid oxygen that allows patients to move more freely; liquid oxygen becomes gaseous when it is warmed

Below is a list of oxygen delivery devices:
- Nasal cannula: soft plastic tubing that is connected to an oxygen source and inserted into the nostrils
- Face mask: plastic mask that covers the nose and mouth and delivers oxygen; delivers more oxygen than nasal cannulas; useful for patients that breathe through the mouth; never removed the face mask without first asking a nurse

Mechanical Ventilation

Mechanical ventilators are machines that breathe for a patient that cannot breathe on their own; they push air into and out of the lungs. Patients may need to be put on mechanical ventilation for a variety reasons (head or spinal injury that affect the breathing control centers, neurological disorders, drug overdose, lung damage, etc.). Alarms will sound if the ventilator detects anything amiss; check that tubes are connected to the ventilator and immediately notify the nurse.

Most patients on mechanical ventilation will also be intubated with an endotracheal tube which means the patient will not be able to speak, drink, or eat. Many patients will also have their wrists restrained to prevent them from pulling out the endotracheal tube.

If patients are to be on mechanical ventilation for more than a week, they will likely need a tracheostomy.

Tracheostomies

A tracheostomy is a surgically created opening into the trachea. Tracheostomies may be temporary or permanent (larynx is removed). Some patients may be able to breathe through the trach without a ventilator, but if a ventilator is needed, a tracheostomy tube is inserted into the opening and attached to a ventilator. Tracheostomy tubes are usually more comfortable than endotracheal tube because it allows patients to eat and drink; some tubes may even allow patients to speak. The tracheostomy tube must be secured to the patient because the tube can be coughed out. For an adult, you should be able to insert a finger under the tracheostomy tie. For a child, you should be able to only insert a fingertip.

Tracheostomy care should be done daily or every 8 to 12 hours. It involves cleaning secretions from reusable cannulas or inserting a new disposable cannula, cleaning the stoma, and applying clean ties or velcro collar.

Never let anything get into the tracheostomy, it can be aspirated into the lungs.
- Cover the tracheostomy to prevent dust, insects, and other small particles from entering
- Do not cover the stoma with non-breathable material (plastic, leather, etc.)
- Be careful when showering, etc. to prevent water from entering the stoma.
- Swimming is not allowed as water will enter the stoma.

Suctioning

Nursing assistants are not responsible for suctioning patients, but are responsible for letting the nurse know when patients need suctioning (noisy breathing, trouble coughing up secretions, etc.) and assisting the nurse as necessary.
Suctioning is done to remove mucus and other fluids from a patient's nose, mouth, pharynx, trachea, and/or bronchi. Because suctioning removes air, along with fluids, the patient can become hypoxic. The different types of suctioning devices include:
- Oropharyngeal suction catheters, such as Yankauer suction catheters, are inserted through the mouth and into the pharynx to suction the mouth and back of the throat.
- Nasopharyngeal suction catheters are passed through the nose and into the pharynx.

Guideline for treating those with respiratory problems (including those on ventilators):
- If oxygen is being used, post an "Oxygen in Use" sign and warn people to not smoke near the area because it can cause the oxygen tank to explode.

- Position patients in the semi-fowler's, fowler's, or orthopneic position for easier breathing.
- If the patient is bedridden, position them to make breathing as easy as possible and change their position every 2 hours because secretions can pool.
- Have patients practice deep breathing and coughing exercises.
- Assist patients with incentive spirometry.
- Observe and record any changes in sputum as it could indicate an infection or other health concern.
- Observe and record changes in breathing patterns. Immediately report signs of difficulty breathing.
- Keeps mouths moist and take care of skin that is in contact with breathing or oxygen delivery devices.
- Maintain proper water levels in oxygen reservoirs to keep delivered air moist.
- Never adjust or discontinue oxygen.
- Never adjust ventilator settings or remove a patient from a ventilator.

Nervous System Disorders

Stroke

There are 2 types of strokes: ischemic and hemorrhagic. An ischemic stroke occurs when a blood clot forms in the blood vessels of the brain, preventing blood flow and causing brain tissue damage. A hemorrhagic stroke occurs when a blood vessel in the brain ruptures or leaks, decreasing blood flow to brain. A stroke on one side of the brain affects the opposite side of the body. Signs and symptoms of a stroke include weakness/numbness in the face and/or limbs, particularly on only one side of the body; facial drooping or drooling; aphasia (inability to speak); nausea/vomiting; lost or dimmed vision; loss of balance; severe headache with sudden onset.

If a person survives a stroke, they may still have permanent damage and loss of function. Patients will tend to "neglect" their weaker side, so it is important that rehabilitation begins as soon as possible.

Parkinson's Disease

Parkinson's is a disease, typically in those over 50, characterized by tremors, stiff muscles, stooped posture and impaired balance, and a blank expression. Over time, the patient will begin to have trouble swallowing and chewing, elimination issues, emotional problems, memory loss, and slower thinking.

Multiple Sclerosis

Multiple sclerosis (MS) is a central nervous system disease where the myelin sheath of the brain and spinal cords are destroyed. Signs and symptoms typically start between the ages of 20 to 40 and include blurred/double vision, muscle weakness, tingling or numbing sensations, partial or complete paralysis, tremors, etc. MS has no cure and patients will often alternate between remission and relapse; eventually symptoms worsen with each relapse.

Amyotrophic Lateral Sclerosis (Lou Gehrig's Disease)

Amyotrophic Lateral Sclerosis is a disease that affects the nerve cells of voluntary muscles. Onset of symptoms usually begins in those between 40 to 60 years of age and most die after 2 to 5 years after onset. Over time the muscles atrophy and patients are unable to control muscles for moving, walking, speaking, chewing, swallowing, and breathing; the patient's intelligence, five senses, and bowel and bladder function usually remain intact.

Brain Injuries

Brain injuries can occur from falls, traffic accidents, sports, etc. Signs of mild brain injury include:
- Loss of consciousness for a few seconds to a few minutes

- Confusion or disorientation
- Headache, dizziness, nausea, or vomiting
- Loss of balance
- Blurred vision
- Ringing in the ears

Signs of moderate to severe brain injury include:
- Signs of mild brain injury
- Loss of consciousness for several minutes to an hour
- Convulsion or seizures
- Dilated pupil in one or both eyes
- Clear fluids draining from the nose or ears
- Inability to wake up
- Loss of coordination
- Slurred speech

Spinal Injuries

Paralysis can result from spinal cord injuries. Depending on the location of the spinal cord injury, a patient may be paraplegic or quadriplegic; the higher the injury is on the spinal cord, the more loss of function. Paraplegics are paralyzed in the legs, lower trunk, and pelvic regions. Quadriplegics are paralyzed in the arms, trunk, legs, lower trunk, and pelvic regions.

Cancer

A tumor is an abnormal growth of tissue. A tumor can be benign or malignant. Cancer is a malignant tumor. Metastasis is when cancer has spread from its primary location to other locations in the body.

One of your roles as a nursing assistant is to notice warning signs of cancer and report it to the nurse. Warning signs of cancer include:
- Changes in bowel or bladder habits, or blood in the stool or urine may indicate color, bladder, or kidney cancer.
- A sore that does not heal may indicate skin cancer. If the sore is in the mouth, it may indicate oral cancer.
- Unusual bleeding or discharge may indicate uterine cancer.
- Thickening or lumps in breast or testicles.
- Enlarged lymph nodes
- Indigestion or difficulty swallowing may be signs of cancer in the digestive system.
- Changes in moles or warts.
- Coughing that doesn't go away; hoarse voice
- Sudden, unexplained weight loss

Treatment of cancer may involve surgery to remove the tumor, radiation, and/or chemotherapy. Patients undergoing radiation may be put under special precautions to prevent exposing others to radiation.

Cancer treatment comes with side effects that you will assist in managing:
- Pain management: notify the nurse if the patient is in pain or there are side effects from pain medications.
- Nausea, vomiting, loss of appetite, diarrhea: provide frequent mouth care; offer ice chips if the patient can't keep anything down
- Radiation therapy may irritate the skin; provide gentle skin care.
- Stomatitis: chemotherapy may cause patients to develop sores in the mouth; provide frequent oral care (use special mouthwash to numb the mouth before providing care)
- Fatigue: mild exercise interspersed with periods of rest help maintain muscle strength
- Increased risk for infections: keep patients away from other people who may have contagious diseases

Lymphatic Disorders

Lymphedema

Lymphedema is swelling in tissues caused by a lymphatic system blockage. It can be painful and limit movement. Elastic garments and bandages are used to help move fluid out and prevent fluid buildup to control swelling. Do not apply a blood pressure cuff on an arm that is at risk for lymphedema (arm in which lymph nodes have been removed).

Lymphoma

Lymphoma is a type of blood cancer. Signs and symptoms include enlarged lymph nodes, fatigue, and weight loss.

Heart Disease

Angina

Angina is chest pain due to reduced blood flow to the heart. Signs and symptoms include pain felt in the chest, shoulders, arms, necks, jaws, or back; paleness; and feeling faint. Resting and nitroglycerin tablets usually help relieve angina. If chest pain lasts longer than a few minutes and is not relieved by rest or nitroglycerin, it may be a signal that the patient is suffering a heart attack.

Atherosclerosis

Arteriosclerosis is a condition that causes the arteries to become more stiff. Atherosclerosis is a form of arteriosclerosis. Atherosclerosis is the buildup of fatty deposits in the coronary arteries (arteries that supply the heart with blood) and is the main underlying condition in patients with coronary artery disease and stroke. The heart may not receive enough oxygenated blood due to the narrowing or blockage of the coronary arteries by fat deposits, blood clots, or spasms. Ischemia (reduced supply of oxygenated blood) leads to tissue hypoxia, which causes angina. If there is inadequate supply of oxygen to the brain, the patient can suffer a Transient Ischemic Attack (TIA). TIAs are similar to strokes except signs and symptoms usually disappear within an hour and always resolve within 24 hours without permanent disability.

Myocardial Infarction

Myocardial infarction is also referred to as a heart attack. Myocardial infarction occurs when parts of the muscles in the heart die due to lack of blood flow and is a medical emergency. Signs and symptoms include sudden and severe chest pain not relieved by rest or nitroglycerin; pain or numbness in 1 or both arms, back, neck, jaws; indigestion; dizziness; nausea; vomiting; cold, clammy skin; fast or irregular pulse; feelings of doom.

Congestive Heart Failure

Congestive heart failure results in a buildup of fluid in the body due to weakening pump capabilities of the heart. Signs and symptoms include edema/swelling of the feet, ankles, and hands; difficulty breathing when lying down; fatigue.

Dysrhythmias/Arrhythmias

Dysrhythmias or arrhythmias are abnormal heart rhythms usually caused by an abnormality in the heart's electrical system. Arrhythmias can range from minor to life-threatening and can be treated through drugs, surgery, pacemakers, or implantable cardioverter defibrillator (ICD). Pacemakers and ICDs are devices that are implanted in a patient to help control abnormal heart beats.

Hypertension

Hypertension means high blood pressure; a patient is considered to have high blood pressure when they have two consecutive readings, in the same arm, over 140/90 mmHg. Chronic hypertension without proper treatment can lead to heart disease and stroke.

Blood Clots

Thrombosis is the formation of a clot in a blood vessel and is considered a medical emergency. Signs and symptoms include a red and warm area in the leg, pain which increases with movement, swelling, etc. Do not massage the leg, ambulate the patient, nor bend the toes upward as these actions can dislodge the clot and cause it to travel elsewhere. Report this to a licensed nurse immediately.

Paralysis

Paralysis may be caused by an injury to the spinal cord; depending on the location of the spinal cord injury, a person may be paraplegic (paralyzed in the lower extremities) or quadriplegic (paralyzed in all four limbs). Hemiplegia is when one side of the body (left or right) is paralyzed. Paralyzed patient are at high risk for contractures, pressure ulcers, respiratory issues, incontinence, and dysphagia (difficulty swallowing).

Guidelines for caring for paralyzed patients:
- Do not continue feeding dysphagic patients until they've completely swallowed the food in their mouth.
- Use thickener with fluids when feeding dysphagic patients.
- Keep dysphagic patients upright for at least 30 minutes after feeding.
- Dress/undress the affected side first.
- When using a cane, a cane should be used on the affected side.
- Perform passive range of motion exercises on all affected extremities.

Digestive Issues

Patients recovering from a stomach infection may be kept NPO (no food or fluids by mouth) and put on IV therapy; only licensed nurses can start, change, and end IV therapy. IV solution bags should be kept above the IV insertion site.

Patients recovering from digestive tract surgery may be kept NPO and may require tube feedings, total parenteral nutrition (TPA) IV therapy, and/or an ostomy (a surgical opening to help in elimination). Feeding tubes, for short term usage, are inserted through the nose and into the stomach. For long term usage, gastrostomy tubes (G tubes) are inserted directly into the stomach through a stoma (a surgically created opening). A diversion is a device attached to a stoma in the abdomen used to eliminate urine. A colostomy is a surgically created opening between the colon and the body's surface that is used to eliminate stool. Depending on where the surgical opening is placed on the colon, stool consistency can range from liquid to formed; the more colon that is left to absorb water, the more solid the stool. An ileostomy is a surgically created opening between the small intestine and the body's surface. Because the entire colon is removed in an ileostomy, stool is not formed/solid; liquid stool drains regularly from an ileostomy.

Gastroesophageal Reflux Disease (GERD)

GERD is a digestive disorder where stomach contents flow back up into the esophagus. Those who are overweight, drink alcohol, pregnant, or smoke are at higher risk for GERD. Signs and symptoms include heartburn, pain in the chest or upper abdomen, sore/hoarse throat, nausea/vomiting, etc. Treatment involves drugs to prevent or reduce stomach acid and life-style changes such as losing weight, quitting smoking, eating smaller meals, staying upright for 3 hours after meals, and wearing loose clothing.

Inflammatory Bowel Disease (IBD)

IBD is a chronic inflammation of the digestive tract. Signs and symptoms include diarrhea, abdominal pain, blood in the stools, loss of appetite, weight loss, etc. Treatment involves drugs to reduce inflammation and pain and diet changes.

Liver Disease

Liver diseases such as hepatitis (viral liver infection) or cirrhosis (scarring of the liver) can lead to liver failure and buildup of toxic waste in the body.

Hepatitis

Hepatitis is a viral liver infection. Signs and symptoms include jaundice (yellowing of the skin or whites of the eyes), fatigue, loss of appetite, pain, nausea/vomiting, dark urine, skin rash, etc.

Hepatitis A is spread through food or water contaminated by the feces of an infected person. People traveling to developing countries, people who live with or sexually involved with an infected person, staff and children at daycares, etc. are at higher risk for contracting Hepatitis A.

Hepatitis B and C are spread through contact with the blood or body fluids of an infected person. Drug users and those sexually involved with an infected person are at higher risk. It may also be passed to a baby during childbirth.

Cirrhosis

Cirrhosis can be caused by chronic alcohol abuse, Hepatitis B or C, and obesity.

Kidney Disease

Kidney diseases can lead to kidney failure and a buildup of toxic waste in the body. It can also lead to heart failure and electrolyte imbalances.

Urinary Tract Infections

Urinary tract infections (UTIs) are common, especially among women. UTIs are usually treated with antibiotics. Signs and symptoms include frequent urination, cloudy or foul smelling urine, pain or burning during urination, etc.

Benign Prostatic Hyperplasia

BPH is prostate enlargement and it is common among older men. As the prostate enlarges, it presses against the urethra, affecting urination. Signs and symptoms include trouble urinating, a weak urine stream, frequent voiding at night, pain during urination, frequent and small voidings, etc.

Kidney Stones

Bedrest, immobility, and inadequate water intake are risk factors for developing kidney stones. Signs and symptoms include severe pain in the back and side below the ribs; pain in the lower abdomen, thigh, and urethra; nausea/vomiting; fever and chills; difficulty urinating; painful urination; cloudy or foul smelling urine; blood in urine; etc.

Kidney Failure

Kidney failure can be acute or chronic. It can take up to a year to recover from acute kidney failure. Hypertension and diabetes are risk factors for developing chronic kidney disease or failure. Treatment for chronic kidney failure/disease includes fluid restriction, diet changes, drugs, and dialysis. Dialysis involves removing waste products from the blood through artificial means.

Endocrine Disorders

Hyperthyroidism (Overactive Thyroid)

Hyperthyroidism occurs when the thyroid gland makes more thyroid hormones than the body needs. People with hyperthyroidism have higher metabolisms. Signs and symptoms include increased hunger accompanied by weight loss, irregular heart beats, insomnia, increased perspiration, and intolerance to heat.

Hypothyroidism (Underactive Thyroid)

Hypothyroidism is the opposite of hyperthyroidism. People with hypothyroidism have lower metabolism. Signs and symptoms include fatigue, weakness, weight gain, constipation, and intolerance to cold.

Diabetes

The body usually uses glucose as a primary source of fuel. Without insulin, glucose cannot enter cells and blood glucose levels will rise. Since the body's cells don't have enough glucose; it begins to break down fat and proteins for fuel. The process of breaking down fat and proteins produces a buildup of acidic ketones in the bloodstream. Since blood glucose levels rise and glucose attracts water, water will leave the cells of the body and lead to frequent urination and dehydration. Dehydration will make a patient feel thirsty and starving cells will make a patient feel hungry. Signs and symptoms of diabetes include frequent urination (polyuria), increased thirst and frequent drinking (polydipsia), extreme hunger and excessive eating (polyphagia), blurred vision, fatigue. Diabetes can lead to blindness, cardiovascular disease, kidney failure, leg ulcers, and nerve damage.

There are 2 types of diabetes: Type 1 and Type 2.

Type 1 diabetes is insulin-dependent and is an autoimmune disorder in which the body attacks the pancreas' insulin producing cells. Patients with Type 1 diabetes don't produce enough insulin, so they require insulin injections to control their blood sugar. Type 1 diabetes is typically diagnosed during childhood or adolescence.

Type 2 diabetes is non-insulin dependent and is typically due to bad lifestyle and diet choices. In Type 2 diabetes, the body is unable to respond to the insulin that is produced.

Glucometers are used to measure blood glucose levels. Normal levels are between 80 to 120 mg/dL. Hypoglycemia is when blood glucose levels are less than or equal to 60 mg/dL. Hyperglycemia is when blood glucose levels are greater than or equal to 120 mg/dL.

Hypoglycemia

Hypoglycemia can occur when a patient takes too much insulin; takes insulin without eating a meal; or takes insulin and eats a meal, but increases physical activity. Hypoglycemic patients may exhibit bizarre and confused behavior. Other signs and symptoms include tachycardia; pale, cool skin; rapid, shallow breathing.

Hyperglycemia/Diabetic Ketoacidosis (DKA)

DKA is a medical emergency where blood sugar levels are high and there isn't enough insulin. Signs and symptoms of DKA include fruity-smelling breath, vomiting, abdominal pain, tachycardia, and unconsciousness.

Guidelines for caring for diabetic patients:
- Snacks in the diet are used to maintain a steady supply of glucose.
- Trim nails accordingly to facility policies; never remove corns or calluses.
- Inspect the skin daily, especially the feet, for signs of pain or decreased sensations which indicate neuropathy, redness, or skin sores which may indicate poor circulation.
- Avoid pressure on feet.

HIV/AIDS

Patients with Human Immunodeficiency Virus (HIV) and/or Acquired Immunodeficiency Syndrome (AIDS) have weakened immune systems, so they must be kept away from patients that are sick. HIV is transmitted through contact with infected blood or bodily fluids so healthcare workers must follow protocol for handling blood and body fluids.

HIV Prevention

- Practice safe sexual behaviors. Anal sex is riskiest, followed by vaginal and then oral sex.
- See a doctor within 3 days of possible HIV exposure for post-exposure prophylaxis.
- HIV negative patients should take pre-exposure prophylaxis (PrEP) drugs if they are involved in a sexual relationship with an HIV positive person or someone at high risk for HIV (gay or bisexual men, drug users, etc.)

HIV Stages

- Acute infection
  - Occurs within 2 to 4 weeks of HIV infection
  - Flu-like symptoms that last a few days to several weeks
- Clinical Latency Stage
  - No to mild HIV related symptoms
  - Lasts an average of 10 years
- AIDS

- o Patient is at risk for pneumonia, TB, Kaposi's sarcoma, nervous system disorders, dementia
- o Signs and symptoms include rapid weight loss, recurring fever, night sweats, sores, fatigue, skin blotches, memory loss, loss of coordination, paralysis

Shingles

Shingles is viral disease characterized by itchy and painful skin rashes with blisters; it is most common in those over 50 years old. It is caused by the same virus as chickenpox and is contagious until the shingle lesions crust over. Shingles are treated with antiviral drugs and take 3 to 5 weeks to heal.

Vision Impairment

Common causes of eye disorders include:
- Conjunctivitis ("Pink Eye"): a highly contagious infection of the conjunctiva (clear membrane that lines the surface of the eye). Signs and symptoms include red, itchy eyes and white or yellow discharge.
- Glaucoma: disease where there is excessive pressure in the eye; it can lead to blindness
- Cataracts: clouding of the lens that can impair vision
- Macular degeneration: causes loss or blurred center vision while leaving peripheral in tact
- Diabetic retinopathy: a complication of diabetes; caused by hardened arteries and damage to the retina

When working with patients that are visually impaired:
- Keep rooms uncluttered and tell patients about where furniture and other things are placed.
- Maintain adequate lighting and to reduce glare, keep light sources behind the patient instead of behind you. Ensure that patients can locate and touch the light before leaving the room.
- Before entering a room, identify and announce your presence. Tell patients when you leave a room.
- Explain any unusual sounds in the room.
- Use the hands of the clock to tell patients about the location of food on the plate.
- Follow facility guidelines for removing, cleaning, and reinserting artificial eyes.

Hearing Impairment

The different types of ear disorders you may encounter include:
- Otitis Media: middle ear infections; chronic ear infections can lead to permanent hearing loss; common in infants and children
- Tinnitus: ringing or buzzing in the ears or head

- Meniere's Disease: fluid buildup in the inner ear that can lead to vertigo, tinnitus, hearing loss

People with hearing impairments find it more difficult to hear high pitch sounds, echos, hollow sounds, fast speech, speech with accents, and when there is background noise.

When working with patients that are hearing impaired:
- Stand in front of patients when speaking to them.
- Talk in a slow and low tone, avoid high pitches.
- Reduce background noise.
- Use sign language, notepads, gesturing to improve communication.
- Ask patients to confirm their understanding of important information by having them repeat it back.

Speech Impairment

Dysphasia or aphasia is a disorder that affects a person's ability to producer and understand speech. Patients with expressive aphasia have trouble expressing their thoughts through speech or writing. Patients with receptive aphasia have trouble understanding language (spoken or written).

Speech impairment can be caused by various reasons ranging from stroke, cancer surgery, Parkinson's disease, etc. Do not try to finish a patient's sentence. Have patients use whiteboards, notepads, etc. to help with communication.

Restorative Skills

The Omnibus Budget and Reconciliation Act requires that long term care facilities help patients maintain their independence and physical and psychological well-being. Patients should be allowed to make their own decisions regarding their life and routine whenever possible.

Rehabilitation is care, provided by a physical therapist, to restore a patient to the highest level of functioning possible. Restorative care, often provided after rehabilitation, is ongoing and includes physical, emotional, and psychological care to help maintain a patient's functioning; CNAs provide restorative care. As a nursing assistant, you duties in rehabilitation and restorative care include:

- Encouraging patients to practice skills and techniques they learned during rehabilitation
- Observe the patient for any changes related to rehabilitation and restorative care
- Providing emotional support

A key part of restorative care is prevention; observing changes and reporting them allows for prompt intervention to prevent disease or disability. Examples of preventative activities include:

- Encouraging patients to walk.
- Feeding patients or encouraging patients to eat to maintain nutrition.
- Turning immobile patients to prevent pressure ulcers.

Physical Therapy

Physical therapy is used to help a patient gain or maintain a person's ability to move and prevent complications from the loss of a function. It usually involves exercise combined with supportive devices (splints, braces, etc.), assistive devices, and prosthetic devices.

Occupational Therapy

Occupational therapy is used to help a patient gain or maintain the skills needed for activities of daily living. It often focuses on improving fine motor skills used for eating with utensils, brushing the teeth, etc.

Speech Language Pathology

Speech language pathology focuses on restoring a patient's ability to speak, chew, or swallow.

Vocational Rehabilitation

Vocational rehabilitation is used to help a patient regain skills needed for their job (vocation).

Mobility

Patients that are immobile are at higher risk for the following:

- Increased risk of blood clots and edema in the lower extremities.
- Decreased appetite which can lead to constipation or anorexia
- Loss of calcium and weaker bones, leading to osteoporosis.
- Muscle atrophy (wasting) and contractures
- Pressure ulcers
- Feelings of social isolation and depression
- Loss of self esteem

To help patients maintain mobility:
- Have patients perform range of motion (ROM) exercises to move all limbs and joints. If patients are unable to perform ROM exercises, perform passive range of motion exercise (PROM) on the patient.
- Teach patients how to use transfer boards to transfer to and from wheelchairs, beds, tubs, toilets, vehicles, etc.

When helping stroke patients walk, stand on their weakest or affected side.

Psychosocial Care Skills

Psychosocial health (emotional and mental well-being) is just as important as physical health. Psychological problems can also put patients in physical danger.

Emotional and Mental Health Needs

As people age, they may be at higher risk for depression stemming from life changes such as losing loved ones, losing independence, etc. Elders who have lost a spouse are at higher risk for suicide because their depression may often go unnoticed.

It is important that you treat patients with respect and care. To show your respect, call patients by their name and title instead of "Honey" or "Sweetie". Show care by spending time, showing interest, and listening to patients. Encourage social interactions and patient participation in their care to promote a sense of independence.

Spiritual and Cultural Needs

If possible, take into account patients cultural background when providing care for them.

Spirituality is often linked with organized religion, but it does not have to be. Patients should have the freedom to practice what they believe in. If you are uncomfortable with a patient's religious practices, tell a licensed nurse so that accomodations can be made.

Sexuality

Patients have a right to their sexual feelings and must given privacy and opportunity to express those feelings appropriately. Unwanted sexual behavior towards another patient or staff member must be stopped and reported to your supervisor.

Sexual Orientation

Sexual orientation refers to the gender a person is attracted to.
- Heterosexuals are attracted to members of the opposite sex.
- Homosexuals are attracted to members of the same sex
- Bisexuals are attracted to members of both sex

Gender Identity

Transgenders or transsexuals have a gender identity that is different from the sex they were assigned at birth. Transvestites dress and behave like the opposite sex for emotional and sexual reasons.

Confusion

Confusion can be caused by physical or psychological factors such as drug side effects, hypoxia, stress, change in routines, etc. Sundowner's Syndrome is a phenomenon where patients become more confused in the late afternoon or early evening. Signs and symptoms of confusion include repeating stories, repeating tasks, being suspicious of staff members, becoming frightened and resisting care, etc.

When patients become confused, it is important to use reality orientation to help patients remember who they are, where they are, etc. Keep calendars, clocks, and bulletins with current events around to support reality for the patient. Do not try to reason with the patient as they are unlikely to understand.

Aggression

When patients become aggressive, it is important that you remain calm and alert the nurses. Signs of aggression include jaw or fish clenching, pacing, crying, or yelling.

Guidelines for dealing with aggressive patients:
- Do not argue with the patient; if you can, leave the situation and return later to let them cool off.
- Sit down but, if you must stand, keep an open stance so you can quickly move away from the patient if necessary. Turn your body slightly away from the patient with your arms at the side; keep your hands open and maintain eye contact.
- Do not hit, push, pull, or retaliate against a resident, even if provoked; it may be considered assault.
- Do not ignore a problem; try to find the cause.
- Try to distract the patient.

Dementia/Alzheimer's

Dementia is a group of conditions that involve the long term decline in brain functions such as memory, judgment, comprehension,etc. Alzheimer's disease is a common type of dementia. Patients with dementia may often feel confused, disoriented, frustrated, depressed, etc. They may also hallucinate and become delusional and paranoid. In later stages, patients can become completely incapacitated (unable to recognize others, unable to swallow, incontinent, immobile, etc.)

In the past, reality orientation was used to manage dementia patients to try to reorient them back to reality (the "here and now"). While reality orientation helped with patients experiencing temporary confusion, it was not very effective with dementia patients. Currently, validation therapy is being used to manage difficult behaviors in dementia patients. Validation therapy focuses on acknowledging a person's reality; instead of correcting a person, distract them or redirect the conversation.

Guidelines for caring for those with dementia:
- Maintain routines to avoid confusion and overstimulation
- Use distraction for agitated or wandering residents
- Use validation therapy
- Arrange evening activities to prevent Sundowner's syndrome
- Follow facility policies for locking doors and windows to prevent wandering
- Do not argue or try to reason with a patient as they are unlikely to understand
- Do not ask a patient to explain any problems as they are unlikely to be able to do so
- Try to comfort and reassure patients

Grieving Process

There are five stages to the grieving process:
1. Denial.
2. Anger.
3. Bargaining.
4. Depression
5. Acceptance.

The fives stages of grief might not occur in the exact order listed above and patients may move back and forth between the stages.

Anxiety Disorders

Generalized Anxiety Disorder: characterized by frequent, persistent, and/or excessive worry or fear over everyday events; particularly future events.

Panic Disorder: an intense and sudden feeling of fear or dread; signs and symptoms may include chest pain, shortness of breath, dizziness, impending doom, etc.

Phobias: an intense fear of an object or situation

Obsessive Compulsive Disorder (OCD): disorder in which a person has uncontrollable, reoccurring thoughts (obsessions) and behaviors (compulsions) that he or she feels the urge to repeat over and over.

Post Traumatic Stress Disorder (PTSD): disorder that develops in some people who have experienced a shocking, scary, or dangerous event.

Depression

Depression is a disorder characterized by a persistent depressed mood and lost of interest in daily activities. Depression can be short term or chronic. Symptoms include insomnia or excessive sleeping, extreme sadness, changes in appetite, withdrawing from social activities, feelings of hopelessness, etc. Severe depression can lead to disability and suicide.

Guidelines for caring for depressed patients:
- Never promise a patient you won't tell others what they say. Although you must keep what a patient tells you confidential, you must report any signs of suicidal ideation (thoughts of committing suicide).
- Watch for statements such as "life is not worth living", "everybody would be better off without me"; these statements may indicate a patient is depressed.
- Encourage them to express their feelings, to be physically active, and to socialize.
- Remove potential hazards in the environment that could be used by patients to harm themselves (razors, belts, etc.)
- Do not make judgmental statements.

Bipolar Disorder

Bipolar disorder, also called manic depression, is a mental disorder that causes extreme mood swings that include emotional highs (mania or hypomania) and lows (depression).

Schizophrenia

Schizophrenia is a mental disorder that may include
- Psychosis (losing touch with reality)
- Hallucinations
- Delusions (false beliefs), delusions of grandeur
- Paranoia
- Thought disorders (trouble thinking logically, making up words, stops speaking in the middle of a thought)
- Movement disorders (repeated movements, agitated movements, catatonic)

Eating Disorders

Anorexia Nervosa is an eating disorder characterized by abnormally low body weight, intense fear of gaining weight, and distorted body image.

Bulimia Nervosa is an eating disorder characterized by binge eating followed by purging (vomiting, etc.) to avoid gaining weight.

Binge Eating Disorder is characterized by binge eating which is NOT followed by methods to purge; it often leads to obesity.

Intellectual/Developmental Disabilities

According to Arc of the United States, a person has an intellectual disability if they have an IQ below 75, a significant limit in 1 adaptive behavior, and onset before age 18. Adaptive behaviors are skills needed for everyday life. Though people with intellectual disabilities may have trouble learning and thinking, they still have physical and emotional needs, including sexual ones.

Down Syndrome

Down syndrome is a genetic intellectual disability where the patient has an extra chromosome. Those with Down syndrome typically have small heads, slanted eyes, short and wide neck, large tongue, poor muscle tone, etc. Many also suffer from heart defects, thyroid issues, hearing and vision issues, digestive issues, etc.

Autism

Autism is an intellectual disorder that affects social skills and communication; onset is typically seen between the 18 months and 3 years. People with autism have trouble understanding social cues, maintaining conversation and eye contact, show a lack of empathy, prefer to play alone, withdraw from physical contact, throw intense tantrums, repeat body movements, etc.

Cerebral Palsy

Cerebral palsy is a group of movement disorders characterized by poor coordination, stiff/weak muscles, abnormal movements, and tremors; hearing, vision, and thinking may also be affected. Onset is usually before the age of 2.

Spina Bifida

Spina bifida is a birth defect characterized by the incomplete closing of the backbone and membranes around the spinal cord. Those with spina bifida may have paralysis or suffer from bladder, bowel, and mobility problems.

Mothers and Newborns

Infant Safety

- Always keeps one hand on a baby on a raised surface.
- Respond to babies' cries to help them feel secure and safe.
- Do not shake powder directly over a baby; it can get into their eyes and lungs.
- Always use both hands to hold a baby; 1 hand supports the head, neck, and upper back and the other hand supports the legs. Neck support is needed for the first 3 months.
- Place infants on a firm surface to sleep. Do not put pillows, quilts, bumper pads, toys, etc. in the crib; they can suffocate babies.
- Crib sheets must fit snugly and not be plastic; plastic can cling to a baby's face, nose, or mouth and suffocate them.
- Lay babies on their back to sleep; babies can lie on their sides or stomachs if they are awake and supervised.

Alert the nurse if you notice any change in a baby's sleep pattern, cry, appetite, activity or any other signs that a baby may be sick.

Sudden Infant Death Syndrome (SIDS)

SIDS is the sudden and unexpected death in those under 1 years old. The cause of SIDS is unknown, however there are steps that can be taken to reduce the risk of SIDS:
- Babies should sleep in the same room as parents, but not in the same bed.
- Breast feed the baby
- Give the baby a pacifier for sleep.
- Keep babies away from smoke.

Elimination

Meconium is sticky, thick, and dark green stool that babies pass for the first 2 days of birth. Breast fed babies have yellow, soft, and runny stools. Bottle fed babies have yellow to brown stools that are more formed. The number of bowel movements a baby has can vary from 1 to 3 bowel movements a day. Babies typically wet their diapers 6 to 8 times a day. Notify the nurse immediately if a baby has diarrhea; diarrhea in babies is very serious.

Umbilical Cord Care

Umbilical cord care is done every time you change a diaper and continues to be done until 2 days after the cord falls off; it takes about 2 weeks for the cord to fall off. Care for the cord by doing the following:

- Keep the stump dry (it should never get wet) and above the diaper
- The baby should be given sponge baths until the cord falls off, after which the baby can be given tub baths.
- Never pull on the cord.
- Report signs of infections (swelling, redness, odor, drainage, bleeding, fever, pain when skin near cord is touched)

Circumcision Care

Circumcision is the removal of foreskin from the penis.
- Clean the penis with every diaper change.
- Use a cotton tip to apply petroleum jelly to the penis.
- Apply the diaper loosely to avoid irritating the penis.

Bathing

Infants are bathed about 3 times a week. They are given sponge baths until the umbilical cord falls off; thereafter, they are given tub baths. To give a baby a tub bath:

1. Fill a bath basin with 1 to 2 inches of water. The water temperature should be between 100F and 105F.
2. Keeping a firm grip on the baby, place the baby in the bath basin.
3. Shampoo and rinse the hair.
4. Use a washcloth with soap formulated for infants to wash the baby's face and then body.
5. Rinse and dry the baby.

Breast Feeding

Babies are fed whenever they are hungry; this is typically every 2 to 3 hours for the first month. Breast-fed babies are nursed more often because breast milk is digested faster. Assist mothers with nursing:

- Have the mother hold the baby in the cradle, side-lying, or football hold position.
- Have the mother stroke the baby's cheek or lower lip with her nipple to stimulate the rooting reflex.
- Make sure the baby's nose is not blocked
- Have her insert a finger into the corner of a baby's mouth to remove the baby from the breast.
- Help prevent dry and cracked nipples by doing the following:

- o   Allow milk on nipple to air dry after feeding
- o   Do not use soap to clean breast or nipples
- Assure mothers that cramping pains in the lower abdomen during breastfeeding is normal

Postpartum Care

Lochia

After delivery, the mother will have vaginal discharge called lochia. Foul smelling lochia is a sign of infection.

- Rubra lochia: bright red discharge that lasts for 2 to 3 days after delivery
- Lochia serosa: pink or brown tinged discharge that lasts for until about 10 days after delivery; report any large clots.
- Lochia alba: white to yellowish discharge that lasts for until about 14 days after delivery

Episiotomy Care

An episiotomy is a cut made in the perineum to make the vaginal opening larger. If the mother had an episiotomy, she will likely find it uncomfortable to sit. Ice may be applied immediately after delivery to prevent swelling. Sitz bath may be ordered for comfort and hygiene.

Admissions, Transfers, and Discharges

Admissions

The admissions process usually starts at the admissions office where patient identification information is obtained and legal documents are signed. The admissions office usually tells the nursing unit when to expect a patient and what room and bed number the patient will be in. In long term care facilities, admission procedures are often done 2 or 3 days before a patient is expected to arrive.

Preparing the Room

1. Practice hand hygiene and put on gloves.
2. Gather the following equipments and place them in the room:
   a. Admissions pack (basin, water pitcher, drinking cup, tissues, personal care items)
   b. Vital sign measurement equipment
   c. Bedpan and/or urinal
   d. Patient gowns or pajamas
   e. Anything else the nurse asks you to get
3. If the patient is expected to arrive by stretcher:
   a. Make a surgical bed.
   b. Raise the bed to allow for the transfer of the patient from a stretcher.
4. If the patient is able to walk or is expected to arrive in a wheelchair:
   a. Make a closed bed.
   b. Lower the bed as directed by the nurse.
5. Attach the call lights to the bed linens.
6. Remove gloves and practice hand hygiene.

Admitting the Patient

1. Identify the patient using two identifiers. Verify the information is correct on the admissions form and ID bracelet.
2. Greet the patient and introduce yourself and the roommate.
3. Depending on the patient's condition, either let them stay dressed in their clothing or have them change into a patient gown.
4. Help the nurse with patient assessment by taking vital signs, measuring weight and height, and filling out the admissions form.
5. Give the patient and family information about where things are located, the purpose of equipments in the room and how to use the equipment, visiting hours/policies, etc.
6. Label personal property and help patients put away clothes and items.

Transfers and Discharges

A patient cannot leave without a doctor's order. The nurse will tell you when to start the transfer/discharge procedures and when the patient is ready to leave.

1. Help the patient dress and pack.
2. Tell the nurse that the patient is ready for a final visit. The nurse will provide the patient with discharge instructions, prescription information, and have them sign discharge papers.
3. If the patient is leaving by a wheelchair:
   a. Get a wheelchair for the patient and a utility cart for the patient's belongings, if necessary. Have a co-worker help you with the utility cart.
   b. Wheel the patient to the exit area and lock the wheels.
   c. Help the patient into the car.
   d. Help put the patient's belongings in the car.
4. If the patient is leaving by ambulance:
   a. Raise the bed rails.
   b. Wait for the ambulance attendants.
   c. When the ambulance attendants arrive, transfer the patient onto the stretcher.

Role of the Nurse Aide

Member of the Health Team

CNAs must work under the supervision of a licensed nurse (RN or LPN) or doctor. Job responsibilities may include, but are not limited to:

- Helping residents perform activities of daily living
- Measure and report vital signs (pulse, respiration, blood pressure, temperature), height, weight, changes in patient's condition, etc.
- Instilling enemas; applying non-sterile dressings; admitting, transferring, and discharging patients; etc.
- Lifting and transporting patients
- Helping patients exercise and improve range of motion
- Keeping patient's room and environment clean and safe

State laws vary so know your state laws regarding what procedures a nursing assistant may perform and which procedures they may not perform. Only perform procedures allowed by your state and facility rules.

Other healthcare members you may interact with include, but are not limited to:

- Registered Nurses (RN). RNs are responsible for carrying out medical and nursing plans for a patient. They supervise and assign personal care activities to unlicensed assistive staff members, LPNs, and CNAs.
- Licensed Practical Nurses (LPN). LPNs also carry out medical and nursing plans for a patient, but work under the supervision of a RN.
- Dietician (RD). RDs create diet plans for a patient to ensure they receive proper nutrition.
- Physical Therapists (RPT). RPTs, under a physician's order, work with patients to maintain musculoskeletal function.
- Respiratory Therapists (RT). RTs, under a physician's order, work with patients to improve their respiratory functions.
- Social Workers (LMHP or LSW). Social workers help patients secure social services such as housing, insurance, etc.

Communication

Good verbal and written communication skills are vital to a successful career as a CNA. Good communication skills require active listening; active listening requires that the listener fully concentrate, understand, respond and then remember what is being said, as well as what's not being said. Active listening also involves the listener observing the speaker's behavior and body language.

When communicating with patients:

- Try not to use medical jargon
- Ask open ended questions
- Use phrases that encourage further exploration of thoughts and feelings
- Use interpreters for non-English speakers
- Be aware of cultural norms such as eye contact, personal space, etc.

In addition to communicating with patients, communicating with other health team members is needed to provide coordinated and effective care. Medical records (chart, clinical record) are used to communicate patient information. The following information should be communicated: what was done, what still needs to be done, and how did the patient respond. It is important to document and report your conversations, observations, and measurements of the patient to your supervisors; observed changes in a patient's condition should be reported to your supervisors promptly.

Medical Records

A medical record is a legal document containing information about a patient's condition, treatments, and response to treatments. It typically contains the following information: admission record, health history, graphic sheets, flow sheets, doctor's orders, progress notes, lab results, consultation reports, assessments, etc.

- The admission record is completed when a patient is admitted; it contains identification information, known allergies, medical conditions, emergency contact, etc.
- The health history is completed by the nurse when the person is admitted; it contains information about the chief complaint (reason for seeking treatment), signs and symptoms, past illnesses, allergies, family history, etc.
- The graphic sheet is used to record measurements and observations such as vital signs, intake and outputs, etc; essentially measurements/observations that are made daily, every shift, or 3 to 4 times a day.
- Progress notes contains information about the treatment given and the patient's response to treatment.
- Flow sheets are used to record frequent measurements and observations such bowel movements, feeding status, bathing, and other activities of daily living.

Kardex or Care Summary

The Kardex or Care Summary is not part of the medical record; it's a quick summary of patient information such as diagnosis, treatments, routine care measures, and special needs.

Assignment Sheets

As assignment sheet is used by nurses to delegate tasks to nursing assistants. It also contains the information a nursing assistant needs to provide care to a patient.

End-of-Shift Reports

The end-of-shift reports is given by a nurse to the on-coming shift nurse. It includes information such as the care given, what care should be given, patient's current condition, and changes that are likely to occur.

Client Rights

All nursing homes are required to have written policies on residents' rights and provide them to the residents. The residents' "Bill of Rights" usually include the following:
- Right to know about the facilities services and charges, including those not covered by Medicare or Medicaid
- Right to be involved in their care.
    - Right to know about their own medical condition, unless otherwise directed by a physician
    - Right to refuse treatment
    - Right to choose their own physician and pharmacy
- Right to all information access (medical records, incident reports, etc.)
- Right to manage their own finances
- Right to privacy, dignity, and respect. Caregivers must knock every time they enter the patient's room.
- Right to use their own clothing and possession unless it poses a safety risk
- Right to air grievances without fear of retaliation
- Right to not be discharged or transferred except for medical reasons (to protect themselves or other residents) or non-payment. Residents must be notified 30 days in advance of a transfer or discharge.
- Right to know when visiting hours are; right to refuse visitors; right to communicate confidentially with visitors.
- Right to be free from abuse and restraint (unless restraints are necessary to protect the patient)
    - Examples of physical abuse include rough handling; withholding food; not changing a wet bed; sexual harassment; etc.
    - Signs of abuse include skin tears or bruises; bruises in different stages of healing; frequent crying; fear of touch; refusal of certain visitors; personality changes; refusal to perform ADLs; etc.

All states must also have an Ombudsman program. An ombudsman is state employee or volunteer (not hospital or facility employee) who advocates on behalf of patient care and rights. They monitor nursing care and investigate and resolve issues.

Legal and Ethical Behavior

Healthcare members have an ethical and legal duty to "do no harm" and provide patient confidentiality.

CNAs may be held liable if they perform duties outside their range of care or if they perform duties incorrectly that result in harm to a patient. Below is a list of situations in which a CNA may be held liable:

- Abuse: Threatening or causing physical or mental harm to a patient.
    - Involuntary Seclusion: Isolating patients as punishment
- Aiding and abetting: Participating or observing in an unlawful act and not reporting it.
- Assault: Threatening to touch or attempting to touch a patient without permission
- Battery: Violence toward a patient; assault is the "attempt" to harm a person whereas battery is the assault carried out.
- Defamation: damaging the reputation of someone through slander or libel
    - Libel: making false statements in writing, pictures, broadcasts
    - Slander: make false oral statements
- False Imprisonment: Preventing a patient's freedom of movement against a patient's wishes, with or without force
- Fraud: saying or doing something to trick a person
- Invasion of Privacy: Exposing a patient's confidential information or exposing a patient's body
- Malpractice: When a professional person is negligent
- Neglect: Accidentally or intentionally ignoring a patient's needs, resulting in harm or injury
- Negligence: Omitting care or performing duties incorrectly, resulting in harm to a patient
- Theft

22 Clinical Test Skills

*You can find state specific nursing standards at the Nurse Aide Registries on the National Council of State Boards of Nursing website (https://www.ncsbn.org/725.htm)

Skill 1: Hand Washing

1. Wet hands and wrists with warm water and then apply soap.
2. **Lather all surfaces of wrists, hands, and fingers producing friction, for at least 30 seconds, keeping hands lower than the elbow. Keep fingertips down and lower than the wrist.**
3. Clean fingernails by rubbing fingertips against the palms of the opposite hand.
4. **Rinse all surfaces of wrists, hands, and fingers, keeping hands lower than the elbows and fingertips down.**
5. Use clean paper towel to dry wrist, hands, and fingers, starting at the fingertips.
6. Throw paper towel into trash can.
7. Use a clean paper towel to turn off the faucet.
8. Do not touch the inside of the sink at any time.

Skill 2: Applying Elastic Stockings

1. Have the patient lie in the supine position.
2. Adjust the bed height to a comfortable working position.
3. Turn stockings inside out, at least to the heel.
4. Place the foot of the stocking over the toes, foot, and heel.
5. Pull the top of stocking over the foot, heel, and leg. Avoid forcing or over-extending any part of the leg.
6. **Ensure that there are no twists or wrinkles. The heel of the stocking should be over the heel and the opening in the toe area, if present, should be over or under the toe area.**
7. Return the bed to the low position.
8. Wash your hands.

Skill 3: Assisting With Use Of Bedpans

1. Practice hand hygiene and put on gloves.
2. Adjust the bed to a comfortable working height. Lower the head of the bed so that the bed is a flat as possible or as much as tolerated by the patient.
3. Fan fold top linens down far enough to place the bedpan.
4. Place a protective pad under the patient's buttocks.

5. Adjust gown or garment to expose the buttocks.
6. Have the patient turn or roll so that they are facing away from you and place the bedpan under the patient. A fracture pan might be needed for immobilized patients. Turn/roll them back so they are in the supine position.
7. Remove and discard gloves. Practice hand hygiene.
8. Raise the head of the bed so that the patient is in a sitting position.
9. Give the patient some tissues before leaving the room.
10. When the patient signals that they are done, enter the room. Knock before entering.
11. Practice hand hygiene and put on gloves.
12. Fan fold top linens to the foot of the bed.
13. Lower the head of the bed and ask the patient to raise their buttocks or roll the patient away from the bedpan.
14. Clean the genital area if the patient cannot do so themselves.
15. Remove and discard the protective pad.
16. Remove the bedpan and empty contents into a toilet. Remove one of your gloves if you need to raise the side rails or touch a doorknob.
17. Rinse and disinfect the bedpan. Place bedpan in designated dirty supply area.
18. Remove and dispose of gloves. Practice hand hygiene and put on clean gloves.
19. Help the patient wash their hands.
20. Remove and discard gloves. Practice hand hygiene.
21. Report and record your observations.

Skill 4: Cleaning Dentures

1. Put on gloves.
2. Line the sink with a washcloth to prevent denture breakage in case you drop the dentures. If you don't take any precautions to prevent denture breakage and the denture breaks, you may be charged with negligence.
3. Ask the patient to take off their dentures. If they need help:
    a. Have them open their mouth.
    b. Hold a gauze between your index and thumb, grasp the upper dentures and move it up and down slightly to break the seal. Remove the dentures and put it in the kidney basin.
    c. Hold a gauze between your index and thumb, grasp the lower dentures, turn them slightly and lift them out. Put the dentures in the kidney basin.
4. Holding the dentures over the sink, rinse the dentures before brushing. Use a denture brush, a toothette, or washcloth and tepid water to clean the dentures. Hot water can warp the dentures. Brush and rinse all surfaces of the dentures.
5. If dentures are to be stored:
    a. Put dentures in a denture cup with water and an effervescent denture tablet and return the covered denture cup to the patient's bedside table.
    b. Use a toothbrush or swab to wash the patient's mouth. Rinse the mouth.
6. If dentures are to be reinserted:

    a. Use a toothbrush or swab to wash the patient's mouth. Rinse the mouth.

    b. Hold the upper dentures using your index and thumb, lift the patient's upper lip, and insert the dentures.

    c. Hold the lower dentures using your index and thumb, pull down the patient's lower lips, and insert the dentures.

7. Wipe the patient's mouth.
8. Report any bleeding or sores to the nurse.

Skill 5: Provide Mouth Care

1. Have the patient sit at a 75 to 90 degree angle
2. Place a towel across the patient's chest to protect the patient's clothing.
3. Perform hand hygiene and put on gloves.
4. Moisten toothbrush with water and then apply toothpaste.
5. **Brush all surfaces of the teeth, tongue, and gums.**
6. Hold emesis basin near the patient's chin and have the patient rinse their mouth. If they are unconscious or unable to rinse independently, use a swab to apply mouthwash to the gums, tongues, and mucous membranes in the mouth.
7. Floss the teeth (optional).
8. Wipe the mouth dry and remove the towel from the patient's chest.
9. Put used linens in the soiled linen hamper.
10. Rinse toothbrush and empty, rinse, and dry the basin.
11. Remove gloves and wash hands.
12. Report any bleeding or mouth sores to the nurse.

Skill 6: Taking The Radial Pulse

1. Have the patient sit or lie down.
2. If the patient is lying down, place their arm straight at their side or fold their arm over the chest. If the patient is sitting down, have them place their arm on a flat surface or support their arm with your arms.
3. Place your first two fingers on the thumb side of the patient's wrist.
4. Note if the pulse is strong or weak and regular or irregular.
5. Count the pulse for 30 seconds and multiply by 2. If the patient has heart disease or the pulse rate is irregular or less than 60 beats per minute, count the pulse for 60 seconds..
6. If the pulse rate is less than 60 BPM or greater than 100 BPM, notify the nurse.
7. Wash hands.
8. Record the rate, strength, type of pulse taken, and regularity of the pulse rate.

Skill 7: Counting Respirations

1. Have the patient sit or lie down.

2. Place your hand on the patient's chest or upper abdomen.
3. Count breaths for 1 minute. One inhale plus one exhale equals one breath.
4. Wash hands.
5. Record the rate, depth, and ease of breathing.

Skill 8: Measure And Record Manual Blood Pressure

1. Let the patient rest for 5 minutes before taking their blood pressure. Tell them to not talk because talking can raise the blood pressure.
2. Have the patient sit or lie down. If sitting, patients should have both feet flat on the ground. The patient's arms should be at the heart level or below if sitting; if lying down, the patient's arms should be at their side. Palms should be up.
3. Check that the manometer reads "0" when there is no air in the cuff.
4. Choose the proper cuff size; a cuff that is too small will result in a higher reading, a cuff that is too large will result in a lower reading.
5. Place the cuff, two finger widths above the elbow, around the patient's bare arms; clothing can affect blood pressure readings because they distort the Korotkoff sounds (blood flow sounds).
6. Place the stethoscope diaphragm over the brachial artery (in the bend of the elbow). Do not place it under the cuff.
7. Close the cuff pump valve and inflate the cuff until you can't hear the pulse. This is the systolic pressure.
8. Continue to inflate the cuff 30 mmHg more and then slowly release the pressure valve at a rate of 2 to 3 mmHg/second.
9. When you hear the first pulse sound, note the reading on the manometer; this is the systolic pressure. Continue listening until the you hear nothing; note the reading on the manometer, this is the diastolic pressure.
10. Wash hands.
11. Record blood pressure.

Skill 9: Putting On And Removing PPE

Putting On PPE

1. Remove watch and all jewelry.
2. Wash and dry hands.
3. Put on a gown with the opening at the back; tie the neck and waist strings. Make sure the gown is snug and covers your uniform.
4. Put on a mask or respirator. Place the mask so that it covers your nose and mouth; tie the mask at the back of your head.
5. Put on goggles or a face shield.

6. Put on gloves. Make sure that the glove cuffs cover the gown cuffs.

Removing PPE

1. **Before removing gown, remove gloves. Remove the first glove by grabbing the glove from the outside and turning it inside out. Use two ungloved fingers to reach inside the other glove and turn it inside out. Throw away the gloves.**
2. Wash hands.
3. Remove goggles or face shield. Lift the headbands to remove the goggles or face shield; do not touch the front of goggles or face shield. The front of goggles/masks are considered contaminated.
4. Remove the gown. Do not touch the outside of the gown.
   a. Untie neck and waist strings.
   b. Without touching the outside of the gown, pull the gown inside out, down, and hold the gown away from you. Do not let the gown touch the floor.
   c. Keep gown inside out and throw it away in a biohazardous waste container; do not put it on the floor.
5. Remove the mask. Untie the strings and remove the mask by grasping only the ties. Throw away the mask.
6. If a respirator was worn, remove the respirator after leaving the room.
7. Wash hands.

Skill 10: Give Modified Bed Baths

1. Perform hand hygiene and put on gloves.
2. Adjust the bed to a comfortable working level. Lock the wheels.
3. Cover the patient with a bath blanket and remove top linens.
4. Help the patient undress and put garments in soiled linen container.
5. Fill a wash basin with warm water (110F to 115F). Add no-rinse cleansing solution if being used. Ask the patient to check the water temperature.
6. Wash hands and put on clean gloves
7. Position the patient in Fowler's position or have them sit at the bedside.
8. The face, hands, underarms, backs, buttocks, and perineal area are washed for a partial bath.
9. **Beginning with the eyes, wash eyes with a wet washcloth (no soap) from the inner eye to outer eye. Use a clean area of the washcloth for each stroke. Wash the face.**
10. Dry the patient's face with a dry cloth.
11. Expose one arm. Place a bed protector or bath towel under the patient's arm to keep the bed dry.
12. Apply soap to a wet washcloth. Wash fingers, underneath fingernails, hand, arm, and underarm, keeping the rest of the body covered. Rinse and pat dry.
13. See "*Giving Complete Bed Baths*" section for instructions on how to wash other parts of the body.

14. Remove and discard gloves. Practice proper hand hygiene and put on new gloves.
15. Give an optional back massage.
16. Apply lotion, deodorant, etc. as requested or ordered.
17. Help the patient dress.
18. Remove and dispose gloves.
19. Report and record any observations.

Skill 11: Dress Patients Who Have An Affected (Weak) Arm

1. Adjust the bed to a comfortable working position. Lower the side rail nearest you.
2. Perform hand hygiene and put on gloves.
3. Cover the patient with a bath blanket. Pull top linens down to the foot of the bed.
4. Help the patient undress.
   a. If the garment fastens in the back:
      i. Lift the head and shoulders or turn the patient so that they are facing away from you.
      ii. Undo buttons, zippers, ties, etc.
      iii. Slide the garment from the shoulder down to the arm. If the patient is on their side, remove clothing from one side, turn the patient on their other side, and remove clothing. **Always remove clothing from the weak or paralyzed limb last.**
   b. If the garments fastens in the front:
      i. Undo buttons, zippers, ties, etc.
      ii. Slide the garment down from the shoulder to the arm, on the strongest side.
      iii. Lift the head and shoulders, bring the garment over to the weak side, and remove the garment.
      iv. If you cannot lift the patient's head and shoulders, turn the patient so they are lying on their weak side, tuck the removed half of garment under the patient. Turn the patient so that they are lying on their strong side, remove garment from the weak side.
   c. If removing a pullover garment:
      i. Undo buttons, zippers, ties, etc.
      ii. Remove the garment from the strong side.
      iii. Lift the head and shoulders or turn the patient so they are lying on their weak side.
      iv. Bring the garment up to the neck and then over the head.
      v. Remove the garment from the patient's weak side.
   d. If removing underwear or pants:
      i. Remove footwear and socks.
      ii. Undo buttons, zippers, ties, belts, etc.
      iii. Ask the person to lift their buttocks. Slide underwear and pants down over hips and buttocks. Lower the buttocks.

iv.   If the patient cannot lift their buttocks, turn the patient so that they are lying on their weak side. Slide underwear and pants, on the string side, off the hips and buttocks. Turn the patient so that they are lying on their strong side; slide underwear and pants, on the weak side, off the hips and buttocks.

v.   Slide underwear and pants down the legs and feet.

5. Help the patient dress. **Always put garment on affected (weak) side first.**

a. Putting on garments that open in the back:

i.   Slide garment onto arm and shoulder of the weak side.

ii.   Slide garment onto arm and shoulder of the strong side.

iii.   Lift the patient's head and shoulders. Button, zip, tie, etc. the back.

iv.   If you cannot lift the patient's head and shoulders, turn the patient so they are lying on their strong side. Button, zip, tie, etc. the back.

b. Putting on garments that open in the front:

i.   Slide garment onto arm and shoulder of the weak side.

ii.   Lift the patient's head and shoulders. Bring garment around to the strong side and return the patient to the supine position. Guide the strong arm into the sleeve.

iii.   If you cannot lift the patient's head and shoulders, turn the patient so that they are lying on their strong side. Place the garment so that it covers the back. Turn the patient so that they are lying on their weak side. Pull the garment out from underneath them. Position the patient so they are lying on their back. Guide the strong arm through the sleeve.

iv.   Button, zip, tie, etc.

c. Putting on pullover garments:

i.   Gather the top and bottom of the garment together at the neck opening.

ii.   Pull the garment over the patient's head.

iii.   Slide the weak arm through the sleeve.

iv.   Slide the strong arm through the sleeve.

v.   Lift the patient's head and shoulders and pull the garment down.

vi.   If you cannot lift the patient's head and shoulders, turn the patient so they are lying on their strong side. Pull the garment down on the weak side. Turn the patient so that they are lying on their weak side. Pull the garment down on the strong side.

d. Putting on underwear or pants:

i.   Slide underwear or pants over feet and up the legs.

ii.   Ask the person to raise their hips and buttocks.

iii.   Bring underwear or pants up over the buttocks.

iv.   If the patient cannot raise their hips or buttocks:

1. Turn the patient onto their strong side and pull underwear or pants, on the weak side, over the buttocks.

2. Turn the patient onto their weak side and pull underwear or pants, on the strong side, over the buttocks.

          v.   Button, zip, tie, buckle, etc. pants.

6. Gather soiled garments and put them in the hamper.
7. Remove and dispose gloves. Practice hand hygiene.
8. Record and report any observations.

Skill 12: Feed Patients Who Cannot Feed Themselves

1. Before feeding the patient, check the name of the meal tray and ask the client to state their name.
2. **Ensure the client is in a sitting position (75 to 90 degrees).**
3. Place the tray in front of the patient.
4. Clean the patient's hand.
5. Sit in a chair, facing the patient.
6. Tell the patient what foods and drinks are on the tray and ask them what they would like to eat first.
7. Offer one bite of each type of food, telling the patient what is in each bite.
8. Offer beverages to the patient throughout the meal.
9. Before offering the next bite or sip, ask the patient if they are ready for the next bite/sip.
10. At the end of the meal, clean the patient's hands and mouth.
11. Remove food tray.
12. Leave patient in a sitting position (75 to 90 degrees).
13. Wash hands.

Skill 13: Position Patients On Their Side

1. Perform hand hygiene and put on gloves.
2. Lower the head of the bed and raise side rail on side to which body will be turned.
3. Help the patient roll onto their side toward the raised side rail.
4. Place or adjust the pillows under the head.
5. Move the patient's arm and shoulder so that the patient is not lying on their arm.
6. Place a supportive device behind the client's back, on the top arm, and between the legs, with the top knee flexed. Support the knee and ankle.
7. Lower the bed.
8. Remove gloves and wash hands.

Skill 14: Measure And Record Urinary Output

1. Put on gloves before handling bedpan.
2. Bring the bedpan to the toilet and pour the contents of the bedpan into the measuring container.
3. Rinse the bedpan and pour the rinse into the toilet.

4. Measure the urine at eye level with the container on a flat surface. If the urine is between measurement lines, round up to the nearest 25 ml/cc.
5. Empty the contents of the measuring container into the toilet.
6. Rinse the measuring container and pour the rinse into the toilet.
7. Remove gloves and wash hands.
8. Record output.

Skill 15: Measure And Record Weight Of Ambulatory Client

1. Ensure the patient has non-skid shoes/footwear on.
2. Ask the patient to empty their bladder.
3. Move the lower and upper weights to 0.
4. Ask the patient to stand on the scale; do not allow them to hold on to you or anything else.
5. Move the upper and lower weights until the balance pointer is in the middle. Note the patient's weight.
6. Wash hands.
7. Record weight.

Skill 16: Perform Modified Passive Range Of Motion For One Knee And One Ankle

1. Perform hand hygiene and put on gloves.
2. Have the patient lie on their back and tell them to tell you if they are in pain.
3. Adjust the bed to a comfortable working height and lock the wheels.
4. **Support the leg at the knees and ankles. Bend and straighten the knees at least 3 times (stop if the patient complains of pain).**
5. **Support the foot and ankle. Turn the foot upward and downward (toes pointing down) at least 3 times (stop if the patient complains of pain).**
6. Lower the bed.
7. Wash hands.

Skill 17: Perform Modified Passive Range Of Motion For One Shoulder

1. Perform hand hygiene and put on gloves.
2. Have the patient lie on their back and tell them to tell you if they are in pain.
3. Adjust the bed to a comfortable working height and lock the wheels.

4. **Support the arm at the elbow and wrist. Raise the patient's straight arm over the head and then lower it. Do this at least 3 times, stop if the patient complains of pain.**
5. **Support the arm at the elbow and wrist. Move the patient's straight arm away from the side of the body to shoulder level and then return towards the body. Do this at least 3 times, stop if the patient complains of pain.**
6. Lower the bed.
7. Wash hands.

Skill 18: Provide Catheter Care

1. Practice hand hygiene and put on gloves.
2. Provide patient privacy and adjust the bed to a comfortable height. Lock the wheels.
3. Fill a wash basin with warm water (110F to 115F) and place it, along with soap, towels, and washcloths, next to the bed.
4. Cover the patient with a bath blanket and fan fold top linens to the foot of the bed.
5. Place waterproof pad under the patient's buttocks.
6. Expose the perineal area.
7. Ask the patient to spread their legs and bend their knees.
8. Check the drainage tubing for any kinks.
9. Provide perineal care.
10. Wet another clean washcloth and apply soap.
11. **Hold the catheter at the meatus (near urethra opening) and continue to hold it there throughout the procedure to prevent tugging the catheter.**
12. **Clean the catheter from the meatus down the catheter at least 4 inches. Use circular and downward strokes, moving away from the meatus. Use a clean area of the washcloth for each stroke.**
13. **Use a new washcloth and the same method as washing the catheter to rinse the catheter.**
14. Use a new washcloth to dry the catheter and perineal area.
15. Secure the tubing to the upper thigh and remove the waterproof pad.
16. Remove and discard gloves. Practice hand hygiene and put on gloves.
17. Pull top linens up and remove the bath blanket.
18. Remove and discard gloves. Practice hand hygiene.
19. Report and record observations.

Skill 19: Provide Perineal Care For Female Patients

1. Perform hand hygiene and put on gloves.
2. Adjust the bed to a comfortable working level and lock the wheels.
3. Lower the head of the bed so it's as flat as possible or as flat as the patient can tolerate. The patient should be lying on her back.

4. Fill a wash basin with warm water (110F to 115F). Add no-rinse cleansing solution if being used. Ask the patient to check the water temperature.
5. Lower the side rail on the side you will be working from. Raise the side rail on the opposite side.
6. Cover the patient with a bath blanket and remove top linens to the foot of the bed.
7. Help the patient undress.
8. Help the patient bend her knees and spread her legs to expose the perineal area (only exposing area between hip and knees); if the patient cannot spread her legs enough to expose the perineal area, turn the patient on her side with the knees bent forward to expose the perineal area.
9. Position the bath blanket like a diamond; so that one corner is at the neck and 1 corner is between the legs. Wrap one corner under and around each leg.
10. Put a bed protector under the patient's buttocks to keep the bed dry.
11. Lift the corner of the blanket that is between the legs, to expose the perineal area.
12. Wet a washcloth. Make a mitt with the washcloth. Always wash with a clean area of the washcloth. Apply soap or no-rinse solution to the washcloth.
13. **Clean the vaginal area. Always use a clean part of the washcloth for each stroke.**
    a. **Separate the labia.**
    b. **Clean 1 side of the labia from front to back (top to bottom).**
    c. **Repeat on other side of the labia.**
    d. **Clean from the top of the vulva and stroking down to to the anus.**
    e. **Rinse and dry the vaginal area.**
14. Turn the patient so that they are facing away from you. Adjust the bath blankets so that only the buttocks are exposed.
15. Wet a washcloth. Make a mitt with the washcloth. Apply soap or no-rinse solution to the washcloth.
16. Separate the buttocks and wash from the vagina to the back. Clean one side, then the other side, and then the middle. Rinse and dry.
17. Reposition the patient.
18. Empty, rinse, and dry the basin. Put the basin in the dirty supply area.
19. Remove the bed protector.
20. Remove and discard gloves. Practice hand hygiene and put on clean gloves.
21. Provide clean linens and incontinence products as needed.
22. Remove gloves and wash hands.
23. Report and record any observations.

Skill 20: Provide Foot Care On One Foot

1. Perform hand hygiene and put on gloves.
2. Fill basin with warm water. Check the temperature and ask patient to check the water.
3. Put basin on a protective barrier and in a comfortable position for the patient to put their foot in.
4. Put patient's foot in the water.

5. Apply soap to a wet washcloth.
6. Supporting the ankle and foot, lift foot from water and wash foot (including between the toes).
7. Rinse and dry foot and toes.
8. Apply lotion to the top and bottom of foot. Do NOT apply lotion between the toes.
9. Empty, rinse, and dry basin. Place basin in dirty supply area.
10. Put used linen/washcloth in soiled linen hamper.
11. Remove gloves and wash hands.

Skill 21: Transfer Patients From Bed To Wheelchair Using A Transfer Belt

1. Move the chair or wheelchair next to the patient's bed, on the patient's strong side. The wheelchair should be at the head of the bed and facing the foot or at the foot of the bed and facing the head.
2. **Raise the wheelchair footplates and lock the wheels.**
3. Lower the bed and lock the wheels.
4. Lower the side rail on your side.
5. Help the patient put on a robe and shoes.
6. **Help the patient sit on the side of the bed with their feet flat on the floor.**
7. If using a transfer belt:
   a. Wrap transfer belt around the patient's waist, over clothing.
   b. Instruct the patient to begin standing when you count to three.
   c. Stand in front of the patient, facing the patient.
   d. On the count of three, grab the transfer belt on each side in an upward motion. Stand knee to knee or toe to toe with the patient to maintain stability.
8. If not using a transfer belt:
   a. Place your hands under the patient's arms and around the patient's shoulder blades.
   b. Tell the patient to hold on to the mattress, put feet on the floor, and lean forward.
   c. Put your feet and knees against the patient's feet and knees.
   d. Tell the patient, on the count of 3, to push against the mattress as you lift them to a standing position.
9. Support the patient and help them pivot until the back of the patient's knees touch the chair or wheelchair.
10. Have the patient grasp the arms of the chair and on the count of 3, lower the patient on to the chair.
11. Position their feet on the footrests.
12. Wash hands.

Skill 22: Assisting To Ambulate Using A Transfer Belt

1. Adjust the bed to a safe and comfortable working position. Lock the wheels.
2. **Before helping a patient stand, ensure that the patient is wearing non-skid shoes/footwear and is in a sitting position with their feet flat on the ground.**
3. While the patient is still sitting, wrap the transfer belt snugly around the patient's waist, over clothing. The buckle should be in front and slightly to the side. You should be able to slide an open flat hand under the belt.
4. Tell the patient to begin standing at the count of three.
5. You should stand, facing the client.
6. Count to three to get the client to start standing. On the count of three, help the patient stand by grabbing the transfer belt on both sides and holding the belt from underneath with two hands. Stand knee to knee or toe to toe with the patient to maintain stability.
7. When walking, walk to the side and slightly behind the patient.

Practice Test 1

1. When you notice signs of physical abuse on a patient, you should
   a. Ask the patient about it
   b. Ask the family about it
   c. Report it to the nurse
   d. Record observations in the patient's chart

2. A safety strap on a wheelchair that a patient can unfasten if desired is NOT considered a restraint.
   a. True
   b. False

3. Unless visible blood is present, which of the following is NOT considered to be contagious? Select all that apply.
   a. Semen
   b. Saliva
   c. Sweat
   d. Wound drainages
   e. None of the above

4. You are preparing a room for a patient. The patient is expected to arrive in a stretcher. What type of bed should you prepare?
   a. A surgical bed
   b. A closed bed
   c. An occupied bed
   d. An open bed

5. A patient with an endotracheal tube will be able to do which of the following? Select all that apply.
   a. Eat
   b. Drink
   c. Speak
   d. None of the above

6. When lifting and moving patients, you should ____. Select all that apply.
   a. Face the patient.
   b. Stand behind the patient.
   c. Use your back muscles.
   d. Twist at the waist.

7. You notice spilled water in a patient's room. What should you do?
   a. Call housekeeping

b. Clean up the spill immediately

c. Place a towel over the spill and tell others to avoid stepping on the towel

d. Place a sign to warn others of the spill.

8. You are preparing a room for a patient. The patient is expected to arrive in a wheelchair. What type of bed should you prepare?
   a. A surgical bed
   b. A closed bed
   c. An occupied bed
   d. An open bed

9. When washing your hands, you should _____. Select all that apply.
   a. Keep your fingers below the wrist.
   b. Keep your fingers above the wrist.
   c. Wash at least 1 inch up the wrist.
   d. Apply soap and then wet your hands.

10. What are signs a patient has a complete airway obstruction? Select all that apply.
    a. The patient is coughing vigorously
    b. The patient is unable to cough
    c. The patient is unable to speak
    d. The patient is clutching his/her throat

11. Every evening, a patient becomes confused and starts accusing staff of stealing her personal items, you should:
    a. Calmly explain to the person that no one can steal her items as the items are stored in a secure area
    b. Rationalize with her by telling her that personal items are stored in a secure area and cannot be stolen
    c. Try to distract her
    d. None of the above

12. Which of the following disease is spread through food or water contaminated by the feces of an infected person?
    a. Hepatitis A
    b. Hepatitis B
    c. Hepatitis C
    d. HIV

13. You made an error while filling out a patient's chart, you should:
    a. Erase the error
    b. Use liquid white-out
    c. Cross out the error and write your initials next to it

d. Start a new form

14. Before serving a meal tray to the patient, you should first:
    a. Identify the patient
    b. Check if the patient has any allergies
    c. Check the temperature of the food
    d. Cut the food into bite sized pieces

15. A patient's nasal cannula has shifted and is now blowing air to his cheeks, what should you do?
    a. Notify the nurse
    b. Remove the nasal cannula
    c. Lower the oxygen level so it doesn't blow air to the patient's cheek
    d. Reposition the nasal cannula

16. Which of the below is outside the scope of practice for a nursing assistant?
    a. Bathing patients
    b. Inserting suppositories
    c. Administering cleansing enemas
    d. None of the above

17. Vest restraints are applied so that _____. Select all that apply.
    a. The back of the vest is in front of the patient's chest.
    b. The back of the best is behind the patient's back.
    c. The flaps are crossed in front of the patient's chest.
    d. The flaps are crossed behind the patient's back.

18. A patient drank 5 fluid ounces of coffee for breakfast. How many mL of coffee did the patient drink?
    a. 30 mL
    b. 40 mL
    c. 60 mL
    d. 150 mL

19. A patient on a mechanical soft diet may be served which of the following? Select all that apply.
    a. Scrambled eggs
    b. Oatmeal
    c. Pureed apple sauce
    d. oranges

20. Which of the following are not expected results of administering an enema? Select all that apply.
    a. Abdominal distension

b. Passing large stools

c. Passing gas

d. Passing watery brown fluid

21. A patient suffers a fall while bathing, you should ___. Select all that apply.
    a. Report the incident to the doctor
    b. Report the incident to the nurse
    c. Write an incident report
    d. Do nothing since it was an accident and not your fault

22. Which of the following are signs of depression? Select all that apply.
    a. Insomnia
    b. Increased sleeping
    c. Increase in appetite
    d. Loss of appetite

23. When a patient is in restraints, a nursing assistant should ____. Select all that apply.
    a. Check extremities for proper circulation every 4 hours.
    b. Check extremities for proper circulation every 2 hours.
    c. Document the reasons for restraining the patient in the chart.
    d. Help the patient be more comfortable

24. A patient's beard should be _____. Select all that apply.
    a. Washed daily
    b. Combed daily
    c. Trimmed daily
    d. Only washed when dirty

25. While helping a patient walk, the patients complains of dizziness. You should
    a. Help them sit in a chair and call for help.
    b. Have them sit on the floor and call for help.
    c. Walk them to their room so they can lie down on their bed.
    d. Put a gait belt on the patient so you can transport them to their room

26. A dementia patients keeps trying to leave the facility, telling you that they need to go home to take care of their baby. You should:
    a. Reorient the patient to reality; telling them their "baby" is now 40 years old and can take care of themselves
    b. Redirect or distract the patient with a conversation about babies
    c. Tell them their baby is waiting for them in their room
    d. None of the above

27. A patient keeps trying to remove their breathing tube. You should _____. Select all that apply.
    a. Apply a mitt restraint
    b. Report your observations to a nurse
    c. Adjust the oxygen flow to make the patient more comfortable so they will stop trying to remove the tube
    d. All of the above

28. Sterilization, washing with bleach, and soaking in alcohol are equally effective in killing microbes.
    a. True.
    b. False.

29. Do not take blood pressure in an arm _____. Select all that apply.
    a. that is on the same side as a mastectomy
    b. that has been affected by a stroke
    c. that is injured or malformed
    d. that has an IV in it

30. A patient is unable to walk or bear any weight. What should you use to transfer a patient to from a bed to a chair?
    a. A gait belt
    b. A mechanical lift
    c. A stand assist lift
    d. None of the above

31. When should personal protective equipment be worn? Select all that apply.
    a. Whenever there is blood in the room
    b. Whenever there is a risk of bodily fluids being sprayed or splashed
    c. Whenever caring for a patient with a suspected infectious disease
    d. All of the above

32. When measuring a patient's temperature from the underarms, you are measuring the
    a. Axillary temperature
    b. Tympanic temperature
    c. Oral temperature
    d. Rectal temperature

33. Areas between the fingers and toes should be kept moisturized to prevent skin cracks.
    a. True
    b. False
34. If a patient is falling, you should
    a. Prevent the fall by holding the patient up

b. Ease the patient to the floor

c. Let the patient fall to the floor; your safety is most important.

d. Catch them by their arm to prevent the fall.

35. The patient's "Bill of Rights" includes the right to know visiting hours.
   a. True
   b. False

36. When is it acceptable to use an alcohol based hand rub instead of washing your hands with soap? Select all that apply.
   a. Never
   b. After taking a patient's blood pressure
   c. When changing gloves during a procedure
   d. When hands have come into contact with blood
   e. After eating lunch

37. Pudding is considered a liquid.
   a. True
   b. False

38. You forget to turn a patient over on a regular basis and the patient develops pressure ulcers; you may be found guilty of?
   a. Assault
   b. Abuse
   c. Negligence
   d. None of the above.

39. When recording intake and output, liquids should be recorded using what unit of measure. Select all that apply.
   a. Grams
   b. Cubic centimeters (cc)
   c. Milliliters (mL)
   d. Ounces

40. How long does it take the mouth to return to normal temperature after drinking a hot liquid?
   a. 5 minutes
   b. 15 minutes
   c. 30 minutes
   d. 60 minutes

41. Negligence is
   a. Accidentally or intentionally ignoring a patient's needs, resulting in harm or injury

  b. Omitting care or performing duties incorrectly, resulting in harm to a patient

  c. Participating or observing in an unlawful act and not reporting it

  d. None of the above

42. What is the first step when dealing with a fire?

  a. Move patient out of harm's way

  b. Pull the fire alarm

  c. Extinguish the fire

  d. Close the fire doors.

43. When helping a stroke patient walk, you should stand behind them.

  a. True

  b. False

44. In what order do signs of a pressure ulcer occur?

  a. Blanching, redness, skin breakdown, bleeding

  b. Redness, blanching, skin breakdown, bleeding

  c. Skin breakdown, bleeding, redness, blanching

  d. Skin breakdown, bleeding, blanching, redness

45. When transferring patients from a bed to a wheelchair,

  a. Brace your knees against the patient's knees.

  b. Brace your feet against the patient's feet.

  c. Brace your thigh against the patient's thigh.

  d. Brace your knees and feet against the patient's knees and feet.

46. What is the most important step before performing a procedure.

  a. Identifying the patient.

  b. Practicing good hygiene

  c. Providing privacy

47. What is the difference between assault and battery?

  a. There is no difference.

  b. Assault is threatening to touch or touching a patient without permission. Battery is violence toward a patient.

  c. Battery is threatening to touch or touching a patient without permission. Assault is violence toward a patient.

  d. None of the above.

48. Where is the apical pulse located?

  a. On the wrist

  b. On the underarms

  c. On the apex of the heart

d. On the foot

49. What does NPO mean?
    a. No food or fluids by mouth.
    b. No food by mouth.
    c. No fluids by mouth.
    d. No fluids before surgery.

50. A patient is unconscious but still breathing; the patient has a "Do Not Resuscitate" order. You should continue to provide life saving treatment.
    a. True
    b. False

51. What is considered a normal respiratory rate for an adult?
    a. Less than 10 breaths per minute
    b. Between 12 and 20 breaths per minute
    c. Between 15 and 30 breaths per minute
    d. Greater than 15 breaths per minute

52. A patient is lying on their side. This position is called the
    a. Supine position
    b. Prone position
    c. Lateral position
    d. Fowler position

53. Sundowner's syndrome is a phenomenon where a patient
    a. Becomes more confused during evening hours.
    b. Becomes more lucid during evening hours.
    c. Becomes happier during evening hours.
    d. Becomes hungrier during evening hours.

54. How many mL is 2 ounces?
    a. 30 mL
    b. 60 mL
    c. 90 mL
    d. 120 mL

55. A person who has hypertension
    a. Has a fast heart rate
    b. Has a slow heart rate
    c. Has high blood pressure
    d. Has low blood pressure

56. In post-surgical recovery, how often should the patient be repositioned?
    a. Every 1 to 2 hours
    b. Every 4 hours
    c. Every 30 minutes
    d. Every 15 minutes

57. When washing your hands, you should
    a. Use a clean cloth towel to dry your hands.
    b. Apply soap after wetting your hands.
    c. Apply soap before wetting your hands.
    d. Wash your hands for at least 10 seconds.

58. Use a toothbrush to brush dentures before placing the dentures in a container with an effervescent denture tablet.
    a. True
    b. False

59. A person has just finished exercising and you need to take their blood pressure, you should
    a. Take the blood pressure immediately because blood pressure readings are most accurate when the heart rate is elevated.
    b. Have the patient take 5 deep breaths to normalize their respiratory rate and then take their blood pressure.
    c. Have them rest for at least 5 minutes before taking their blood pressure.
    d. Have them rest for at least 20 minutes before taking their blood pressure.

60. How often should patient intake and output be recorded?
    a. Every 4 hours
    b. Every 12 hours
    c. Every 24 hours
    d. At the end of a shift

61. How often should immobile patients be turned?
    a. Every 2 hours
    b. Every 4 hours
    c. Every 8 hours
    d. Every 12 hours

62. How should you transfer a patient that may have suffered a spinal injury?
    a. Use a mechanical lift
    b. Use a transfer belt
    c. Logroll the patient
    d. Any of the above

63. A patient is weak, but able to walk. What should you use to transfer a patient from a bed to a chair?
    a. A gait belt
    b. A mechanical lift
    c. A stand assist lift
    d. None of the above

64. The perineal area should be cleaned before performing which of the following procedures?
    a. 24 hour urine specimen
    b. Routine urine specimen
    c. Clean catch urine specimen
    d. All of the above

65. When assisting with physical exams, you should stay in the exam room if ___. Select all that apply.
    a. You are female, the patient is female, and the examiner is male
    b. You are male, the patient is male, and the examiner is male
    c. You are male, the patient is female, and the examiner is male
    d. You are male and the female examiner wants you there when examining a male

66. Thin, red-tinged, watery drainage from a wound is called:
    a. Serous drainage
    b. Sanguineous drainage
    c. Serosanguineous drainage
    d. Purulent drainage

67. An abnormal shortening or hardening of muscles is called
    a. Atrophy
    b. Fracture
    c. Sprain
    d. Contracture

68. In post-surgical recovery, how often should you measure a patient's vital signs?
    a. Every 15 minutes until the patient is stable
    b. Every 30 minutes until the patient is stable
    c. Every hour for 4 hours
    d. Every 4 hours

69. What PPE should be worn when changing soiled linens?
    a. Gloves
    b. Gown

c. Goggles

d. Gloves and gown

70. What is a normal resting heart rate?

    a. 50 to 100 beats per minute

    b. 60 to 100 beats per minute

    c. 50 to 120 beats per minute

    d. 60 to 120 beats per minute

Practice Test 1 Answers

1. C. You should report it to the nurse. The nurse is responsible for asking the patient about the possible abuse and documenting it.

2. A. If a patient is physically and mentally able to unfasten a device, that device is NOT considered a restraint.

3. B,C. Unless visible blood is present, the following is not considered to be contagious: feces, nasal secretions, saliva, sputum, sweat, tears, urine,vomitus.

4. A. If the patient is expected to arrive in a stretcher, prepare a surgical bed.

5. D. Patients with endotracheal tubes will not be able to speak, eat, or drink.

6. A. When lifting and moving patients, you should face the patient and keep the patient as close to the body as possible. Use both arms, your legs, hip, gluteal, and abdominal muscles. Do not use your back muscles. Avoid twisting at the waist. When moving the patient's body, move the top first, than torso, and then the legs. In certain situations, you may need to log roll (roll the patient as a single unit, keeping the neck and spine as straight and still as possible) the patient.

7. B. You should clean spills immediately.

8. B. If the patient is expected to arrive in a wheelchair or is able to walk, prepare a closed bed.

9. A,C. When washing your hands, you should wet your hands and then apply soap; keep fingers below the wrist; wash hands for at least 30 seconds; clean the back and front of hands, at least one inch up the wrists, between fingers, cuticles, and under nails.

10. B,C.D. A patient with an airway obstruction will be unable to cough or speak; they are also likely to be clutching their throat.

11. C. Do not try to argue, explain, or rationalize with a patient experience Sundowner's syndrome as they are unlikely to understand. Instead, try to distract or comfort them.

12. A. Hepatitis A is spread through food or water contaminated by the feces of an infected person. Hepatitis B and C and HIV are spread through contact with the blood or body fluids of an infected person.

13. C. Never erase an error. Cross the error out and write your initials next to it.

14. A. Always identify the patient before performing a procedure or serving a meal. After identifying the identity, check for allergies.

15. D. Repositioning the nasal cannula is within the scope of practice for nursing assistants and does not require notifying the nurse. Never remove a nasal cannula or change the oxygen flow rate.

16. B. Suppositories are considered drugs. Administering medication or drugs is out of the scope of practice for nursing assistants.

17. B,C. Vest restraints should be applied so that the back of the vest is behind the patient's back and the flaps are crossed in front of the patient's chest.

18. D. The patient drank 150 mL of coffee. 1 fluid ounce equals 30 mL, so 5 fluid ounces equal 150 mL.

19. C. Patients on mechanical soft diets may only be served food that has been pureed.

20. A. Abdominal distension and pain are signs of enema retention and should be reported immediately to the nurse. Passing formed stools, gas, or watery brown fluid is not unusual.

21. B,C. All accidents and incidents must be verbally reported to the nurse immediately. A written incident report must also be filled out.

22. A,B,C,D. Changes in sleep habits (insomnia, increased sleeping) and changes in appetite are all signs of depression.

23. D. The nursing assistant should help the patient be more comfortable. Nurses, not nursing assistants, check extremities every 4 hours and document the reasons for restraints.

24. A,B. A patient's beard should be washed and combed daily. Beards should not be trimmed unless requested by the patient.

25. A. If a patient complains of dizziness, have them sit in a nearby chair and call for help. If a chair is not nearby, have them sit on the floor.

26. B. Redirect or distract the patient.

27. B. You should report your observations to the nurse. You must not apply restraints unless there is a doctor's order.

28. B. Although washing with bleach and soaking in alcohol does kill some microbes, sterilization is the most effective method of killing microbes.

29. A,B,C,D. Do not take blood pressure in an arm that is on the same side as a mastectomy, that has been affected by a stroke, that is injured or malformed, or that has an IV in it.

30. B. A mechanical lift is used to transfer patients that are too heavy, cannot walk, or unable to help in the transfer. Stand assist lifts are used when a patient is can bear some weight, sit up at the side of the bed with or without assistance, and bend the hips, knees, and ankles. A gait belt is used when a patient is able to walk.

31. B,C. Personal protective equipment should be worn when there is a risk of being sprayed or splashed with bodily fluids or when an infectious disease is suspected.

32. A. The axillary temperature is measured from the underarms. The tympanic temperature is measured through the ears.

33. B. False. Keep the area between fingers and toes dry (avoid lotion) to prevent bacterial growth and skin breakdown.

34. B. If a patient is falling, do not try to prevent the fall; you may injure yourself and the patient. Instead, place your body behind the person and wrap your arounds around the torso; ease the patient to the floor by letting them slide down your body, while protecting their head. Before moving the person, wait for the nurse to assess if the patient is injured.

35. A. All nursing homes are required to have written policies on residents' rights and provide them to the residents. The residents' "Bill of Rights" includes many rights to support their independence and privacy, including the right to know visiting hours.

36. B,C. Alcohol based hand rub may be used when performing routine care procedures where you do not come into contact with body fluids or when changing gloves during a procedure.

37. A. True. Foods that are liquid at room or body temperature (ice cream, gelatin, pudding, etc.) are considered liquids.

38. C. You may be found guilty of negligence. Negligence is omitting care or performing duties incorrectly, resulting in harm to a patient. Assault is threatening to touch or

touching a patient without permission. Abuse is threatening or causing physical or mental harm to a patient.

39. B,C. When recording intake and output, liquids should be recorded in cubic centimeters (cc) or milliliters (mL).

40. B. It takes 15 minutes for the mouth to return to normal temperature after smoking or drinking a hot or cold beverage; this is why you have to wait 15 minutes before taking oral temperatures if a patient recently smoked or had a hot or cold beverage.

41. B. Negligence: Omitting care or performing duties incorrectly, resulting in harm to a patient. Neglect: Accidentally or intentionally ignoring a patient's needs, resulting in harm or injury. Aiding and abetting: Participating or observing in an unlawful act and not reporting it.

42. A. The first step is to move the patient out of harm's way and then pull the fire alarm.

43. B. False. When helping stroke patients walk, you should stand on their weakest or affected side.

44. B. The first sign of a pressure ulcer is redness, then blanching, skin breakdown, and bleeding.

45. D. When transferring patients from a bed to a wheelchair, brace your knees and feet against the patient's knees and feet as you lift them into a standing position.

46. A. Although practicing good hygiene and providing patient privacy are both extremely important, identifying the patient is the most important step before performing a procedure.

47. B. Assault is threatening to touch or touching a patient without permission. Battery is violence toward a patient.

48. C. The apical pulse is located at the apex of the heart. The radial pulse is located on the wrist. The dorsal pulse is located on the foot.

49. A. NPO means no food or fluids by mouth.

50. A. True. "Do Not Resuscitate" orders do not go into effect until a patient is in respiratory or cardiac arrest; until then, continue to provide life saving treatment.

51. B. A normal respiratory rate for an adult is between 12 and 20 breaths per minute.

52. C. In the lateral position, a patient is lying on their side. In the supine position, a patient is lying on their back with their face up. In the prone position, a patient is lying on their stomach with their face down. In the fowler position, a patient is lying on their back with the upper body elevated at a 45 to 60 degree angle.

53. A. Sundowner's syndrome is a phenomenon where a patient becomes more confused during the evening hours.

54. B. 1 ounce is 30 mL, so 2 ounces is 60 mL.

55. C. Hypertension means high blood pressure. Hypotension means low blood pressure. Tachycardia means fast heart rate. Bradycardia means slow heart rate.

56. A. In post-surgical recovery, the patient should be repositioned every 1 to 2 hours to prevent respiratory and circulatory issues.

57. B. When washing your hands, you should apply soap after wetting your hands. Wash your hands for at least 30 seconds and use a clean paper towel to dry your hands.

58. B. Never use a toothbrush to brush dentures; it can scratch the dentures and allow bacteria to grow in it. Use a denture brush, a toothette, or washcloth to wash dentures.

59. C. If a patient was recently active, wait at least 5 minutes before taking their blood pressure.

60. D. Intake and output should be recorded at the end of a shift.

61. A. Immobile patients should be turned every 2 hours. After 4 hours in the same position, skin may begin to break down.

62. C. If a patient may have a spinal injury, you should keep the head, neck, and spine aligned by logrolling the patient.

63. A. A gait belt can be used to transfer patients that can walk. A mechanical lift is used to transfer patients that are too heavy, cannot walk, or unable to help in the transfer. Stand assist lifts are used when a patient is can bear some weight, sit up at the side of the bed with or without assistance, and bend the hips, knees, and ankles.

64. C. The perineal area should be cleaned before collecting a clean catch specimen.

65. A,B,D. When assisting with physical exams, you should stay in the exam room if: you are female, the patient is female, and the examiner is male; you are male, the patient is

male, and the examiner is male; you are male and the female examiner wants you there when examining a male.

66. C. Serosanguineous drainage: thin, watery drainage that is red tinged. Serous drainage: clear, watery fluid; fluid in a blister is serous. Sanguineous drainage: bloody drainage; bright red drainage indicates newer bleeding whereas dark red drainage indicates older bleeding. Purulent drainage: thick green, yellow, or brown drainage.

67. D. A contracture is an abnormal shortening/hardening of muscles that leads to deformity and rigidity of joints.

68. A. In post-surgical recovery, you should measure a patient's vital signs every 15 minutes until the patient is stable, then every 30 minutes for 1 to 2 hours, then every hour for 4 hours, and then every 4 hours.

69. A. Gloves should be worn when changing soiled linens.

70. B. 60 to 100 beats per minutes is considered normal.

Practice Test 2

1. When selecting a site for a skin puncture for blood glucose testing, you should _____. Select all that apply.
    a. Choose the center or fleshy parts of the fingers
    b. Avoid areas with bruises
    c. Avoid areas with calluses
    d. All of the above

2. While performing the Heimlich maneuver, the patient becomes unconscious. You should check if the patient has a pulse before performing chest compressions.
    a. True
    b. False

3. Which of the following statements are true. Select all that apply.
    a. Dry heat penetrates deeper and faster than moist heat.
    b. Moist heat lasts longer than dry heat.
    c. Moist cold applications penetrates deeper and slower than dry cold applications.
    d. Heat and cold applications are applied no longer than 15 to 20 minutes

4. Which of the following is a good source of Vitamin D? Select all that apply.
    a. Leafy greens
    b. Sunlight
    c. Beef
    d. Fish liver oils

5. Which of the following should be done to prevent pressure ulcers? Select all that apply.
    a. Reposition patients at least every 2 hours
    b. Avoid tight clothing
    c. Tell patients to not sit with their legs crossed
    d. Wear well fitting shoes and break in new shoes slowly

6. Casted arms and legs should be elevated to prevent swelling.
    a. True
    b. False

7. When dealing with an aggressive patient, what guidelines should you follow? Select all that apply.
    a. Do not argue with the patient
    b. Ignore the patient

    c. Keep your hands open

    d. All of the above

8. Gloves should be removed before recording a procedure.

    a. True

    b. False

9. You should notify a nurse if a newborn's heart rate is ___. Select all that apply.

    a. 80 beats per minute

    b. 140 beats per minute

    c. 160 beats per minute

    d. 180 beats per minute

10. A patient is complaining of severe pain in the back and side below the ribs, and painful urination. You should report this to the nurse because the patient may be suffering from:

    a. A urinary tract infection

    b. Kidney failure

    c. Kidney stones

    d. BPH

11. A patient who has trouble swallowing is put on a pureed diet. What foods can the patient eat? Select all that apply.

    a. Apple sauce

    b. Mashed potatoes and gravy

    c. Peanut butter

    d. All of the above

12. When administering enemas, what position should the patient be in?

    a. Left Sim's position

    b. Right Sim's position

    c. Semi-fowler position

    d. Prone position

13. Before a resident of a long term care facility can be transferred or discharged, how much notice must they be given?

    a. 24 hours

    b. 7 days

    c. 30 days

    d. 60 days

14. When caring for patients with vision impairment, you should ___. Select all that apply.

    a. Keep light sources behind you.

    b. Identify and announce your presence before entering a room.

    c. Use the hands of the clock to tell patients about the location of food on the plate.

    d. All of the above

15. A patient's input and output totals should be documented in the patient's records
    a. Every 8 hours
    b. Every 24 hours
    c. At the end of your shift
    d. Documenting input and output is not a nursing assistant's responsibility

16. You should notify the nurse if a mother experiences any pain during breastfeeding.
    a. True
    b. False

17. You can share private health information with
    a. A patient's wife
    b. A patient's fiance
    c. The nursing assistant on the next shift
    d. No one

18. What is a normal pulse oximetry reading?
    a. 90% to 100%
    b. 95% to 100%
    c. 80% to 100%
    d. 85% to 100%

19. Which of the following should be included in a patient's intake record. Select all that apply.
    a. An apple
    b. A glass of milk
    c. A granola bar
    d. IV fluids

20. When treating patients suffering from nausea and vomiting, you should ___. Select all that apply.
    a. Serve the patient usual meals in hopes of increasing their appetite
    b. Give them nausea medication
    c. Provide frequent oral care
    d. Offer them ice chips

21. What special care considerations should you provide a patient with hypothyroidism? Select all that apply.
    a. Dress the patient warmly as they are intolerant to cold
    b. Have the patient eat meals and snacks on a regular schedule

    c. Inspect the feet daily for signs of pain or decreased sensations

    d. Have the patient eat lots of fiber as they are likely to become constipated

22. You notice the left side of a patient's face is drooping; this may be a sign of:
    a. A seizure
    b. Aphasia
    c. A stroke
    d. None of the above

23. How often should condom catheters be changed?
    a. Everytime the patient urinates
    b. Once a day
    c. Every 8 hours
    d. Every 2 to 7 days

24. Before death, what is the last sense to go?
    a. Sight
    b. Hearing
    c. Smell
    d. Taste
    e. Touch

25. Before bathing a patient, you should first
    a. Check the water temperature
    b. Gather all the necessary supplies
    c. Have the patient urinate
    d. Check the care plan to see if the patient is allowed to have a bath

26. Which type of catheter should be removed after emptying the bladder?
    a. Straight catheter
    b. Retention catheter
    c. Foley catheter
    d. All of the above

27. When securing a wound dressing, you should apply tape:
    a. Across the top and bottom of a dressing
    b. Across the top, middle, and bottom of a dressing
    c. Diagonally, forming an "X" over the dressing
    d. So it encircles the dressing and body part

28. When collecting a sputum specimen, you should? Select all that apply.
    a. Have the patient rinse their mouth with an antiseptic
    b. Have the patient rinse their mouth with water

c. Have the patient cough deeply for the sputum specimen

d. None of the above

29. When dressing or undressing patients, you should _____. Select all that apply.
    a. Remove clothing from the weak or paralyzed limb last
    b. Remove clothing from the weak or paralyzed limb first
    c. Clothe the weak or paralyzed limb last
    d. Clothe the weak or paralyzed limb first

30. How often should ostomy pouches be changed?
    a. Everytime the patient has a bowel movement
    b. Every 8 hours
    c. Once a day
    d. Every 2 to 7 days

31. Restoration is the care to restore a patient to the highest level of functioning possible.
    a. True
    b. False

32. What special care considerations should you provide a patient with diabetes? Select all that apply.
    a. Dress the patient warmly as they are intolerant to cold
    b. Have the patient eat meals and snacks on a regular schedule
    c. Inspect the feet daily for signs of pain or decreased sensations
    d. Have the patient eat lots of fiber as they are likely to become constipated

33. A patient is having a seizure. You should _____. Select all that apply.
    a. Turn the patient on their side.
    b. Put something in their mouth to prevent them from biting their tongue.
    c. Hold the patient firmly to prevent movements that can cause injury.
    d. All of the above

34. During post-mortem care, the patient's body is put into alignment after rigor mortis sets in.
    a. True
    b. False

35. When using a glass thermometer, you should shake the thermometer until the substance is:
    a. Above the 98.6F mark
    b. Below the 98.6F mark
    c. Above the 94F mark
    d. Below the 94F mark

36. A patient with difficulty chewing may best benefit from:
    a. Physical therapy
    b. Occupational therapy
    c. Speech-language pathology
    d. Vocational therapy

37. Normal glucose levels are:
    a. Between 60 and 80 mg/dL
    b. Between 80 and 120 mg/dL
    c. Below 60 mg/dL
    d. Greater than 120 mg/dL

38. What viral disease is characterized by itchy and painful skin rashes with blisters and most common in those over 50 years old?
    a. Chicken pox
    b. Rubella
    c. Fever blisters
    d. shingles

39. Which of the statements regarding linens is true. Select all that apply.
    a. Hold the linen close to your body
    b. Do not let linens touch the floor
    c. Never shake linens
    d. Fold the soiled side of linens outward

40. You should place wet casts on a hard surface to dry.
    a. True
    b. False

41. A patient having trouble using utensils to eat may best benefit from:
    a. Physical therapy
    b. Occupational therapy
    c. Speech-language pathology
    d. Vocational therapy

42. A terminal patient says that he will believe in God if God will grant him more time. This an example of:
    a. Acceptance
    b. Depression
    c. Bargaining
    d. Denial

43. When providing oral care for an unconscious patient, you should

a. Turn the patient and the patients head to the side
b. Position the patient's head so they are facing the ceiling
c. Raise the head of the bed
d. None of the above

44. People with hearing impairments have trouble hearing high pitch sounds.
    a. True
    b. False

45. When providing male perineal care, clean the penis
    a. From the base to the tip, using circular motions
    b. From the base to the tip, using straight strokes
    c. From the tip to the base, using circulator motions
    d. From the tip to the base, using straight strokes

46. Which of these are signs of impending death? Select all that apply.
    a. Cheyne-Stokes respirations
    b. Increased body movements
    c. Increased blood pressure
    d. None of the above

47. Hypoglycemia occurs when a patient _____. Select all that apply.
    a. Does not take enough insulin
    b. Take too much insulin
    c. Takes insulin without eating a meal
    d. Takes insulin with a meal, but increases physical activity

48. There are 10 mL of water in the balloon of an indwelling catheter, you were only able to draw 9mL out of the balloon, what should you do next?
    a. Since you were able to draw out over 75% of the water in the balloon, you can safely continue to remove the catheter
    b. Squeeze the balloon to completely empty the balloon of water
    c. Pop the balloon to completely empty the balloon of water
    d. Stop and notify the nurse

49. Why should a patient avoid food and fluids before surgery?
    a. To prevent the patient from urinating or having a bowel movement during surgery
    b. To prevent a patient from vomiting and aspirating food or fluids during surgery
    c. Anesthesia is more effective on an empty stomach
    d. All of the above

50. You are caring for a patient recovering from a hip replacement surgery. What should you do? Select all that apply.

a. Remember to exercise the affected leg to maintain flexibility of the leg
b. Remember to externally rotate the hips
c. Have the patient use an abduction pillow when in a supine or lateral position
d. Encourage the patient to try to walk a couple of days after surgery

51. A patient has a musculoskeletal injury. You want to relieve the patient's pain and swelling, you should:
    a. Apply a cold compress
    b. Apply a hot compress
    c. Apply a hot compress to relieve the pain and then a cold compress to relieve the swelling
    d. Apply a cold compress to relieve the swelling and then a hot compress to relieve the pain.

52. A patient has a red and warm area on the leg and complains of increased pain with movement, you should ? Select all that apply.
    a. Massage the leg to help with the pain
    b. Help the patient walk to increase blood flow
    c. Bend the patient's toes upwards to stretch the legs
    d. None of the above

53. Which of the following statements are true. Select all that apply.
    a. A person is only contagious when they have an active TB infection.
    b. Patients with TB cannot be treated in long term care facilities.
    c. You only need to wear a respirator if you are within 10 feet of a TB patient.
    d. TB patients should wear masks when being transported, in waiting areas, and when others are present.

54. As a nursing assistant, your responsibility in rehabilitation and restorative care includes ___. Select all that apply.
    a. Encourage the patient to practice skills they learned during rehabilitation
    b. Report signs of chafing from use of supportive devices
    c. Teach the patient technique to regain chewing abilities
    d. All of the above.

55. For a 24 hour urine recording for an adult, which of these 24 hour urine values are concerning? Select all that apply.
    a. 600 mL
    b. 800 mL
    c. 1500 mL
    d. 2500 mL

56. To show respect and care to patients, you should ___. Select all that apply.

a. Call them "Sweetie", "Honey" or other terms of endearment.
b. Spending time with them
c. Showing interest in them
d. Listening to them

57. A patient believes he is Jesus Christ. This is an example of:
   a. A hallucination
   b. A delusion
   c. Nervosa
   d. A religious episode

58. A patient spills hot tea on her lap. The area is painful and red, but there are no blisters. This is a sign of:
   a. A first degree burn
   b. A second degree burn
   c. A third degree burn

59. After eating dinner, a patient breaks out in hives, this is most likely due to:
   a. An allergic reaction
   b. Eczema
   c. A skin disorder
   d. None of the above

60. Why should coughing and deep breathing exercises be done post surgery?
   a. To prevent circulatory complications
   b. To prevent pulmonary embolisms
   c. To prevent pneumonia
   d. All of the above

61. To avoid pulling a catheter, the catheter should be taped to
   a. The upper thigh
   b. The outer thigh
   c. The hip
   d. The knee

62. MRSA is a
   a. bacterial infection that mainly affects the lungs
   b. bacterial infection of the skin that can spread to the bloodstream
   c. skin infection caused by tiny mites that cause rashes and intense itching
   d. an infection caused by a virus that attacks a nerve path, causing pain and disability

63. Which of the following is not allowed on a clear liquid diet?

a. Water

b. Fat free broth

c. Coffee

d. Orange juice with pulp

64. Canes should be held:

    a. 4 to 5 inches to the side and 4 to 5 inches in front of the strong foot

    b. 4 to 5 inches to the side and 4 to 5 inches in front of the weak foot

    c. 6 to 10 inches to the side and 6 to 10 inches in front of the strong foot

    d. 6 to 10 inches to the side and 6 to 10 inches in front of the strong foot

65. A patient has been diagnosed with a terminal illness. You should:

    a. Avoid bringing up the diagnosis unless the patient brings it up

    b. Offer to contact a pastor or spiritual leader

    c. Share your beliefs of the afterlife with them to give them hope

    d. All of the above

66. When shaving patients on anticoagulants, you should:

    a. Always use a safety razor

    b. Always use an electric razor

    c. Do not shave patients on anticoagulants

    d. Only nurses are allowed to shave patients on anticoagulants

67. A patient is feeling very anxious, how can you help?

    a. Remain calm and comfort them

    b. Leave the patient alone so they have time to calm themselves

    c. Try to distract the patient

    d. All of the above

68. The main benefits of bathing include ___. Select all that apply?

    a. Keeps patients clean

    b. Improves circulation by stimulating the muscles.

    c. Provides exercise for the joints and limbs.

    d. Gives CNAs the opportunity to inspect the patient's skin, mobility, and health.

69. Which of the following is a sign of hepatitis?

    a. Hyperglycemia

    b. Hypotension

    c. Dyspnea

    d. Jaundice

70. When performing abdominal thrusts, where should your fist be placed?

    a. Above the patient's navel

b. Below the patient's navel
c. Right below the patient's chest
d. Both above or below the navel is acceptable

Practice Test 2 Answers

1. B, C. When choosing a site for a skin puncture, avoid areas with calluses (those areas have bad blood flow); avoid swollen, bruised, scarred, or cyanotic areas; do not use sites with many nerve endings which can make it painful (e.g., center or fleshy parts of fingers). Use the side of the middle or ring finger tip

2. B. If the patient becomes unconscious while you are performing the Heimlich maneuver, you should begin chest compressions right away, whether or not the patient has a pulse.

3. D. Moist heat applications (water is in contact with the skin) penetrate deeper and faster than dry heat applications, so lower temperatures are used. Dry heat applications don't penetrate as deep, but the heat lasts longer. Moist cold applications also penetrate deeper and faster than dry cold applications, so higher temperatures are used. Heat and cold applications are applied no longer than 15 to 20 minutes.

4. B, D. Sunlight and fish liver oils are good sources of Vitamin D.

5. A,B,C,D. To prevent pressure ulcers: reposition patients at least every 2 hours; avoid tight clothing; tell patients to not sit with their legs crossed; do not scrub or rub the skin; avoid pressure on the heels of feet and other bony areas; wear well fitting shoes and break in new shoes slowly; use proper protective devices.

6. A. True

7. A, C. Guidelines for dealing with aggressive patients:
Do not argue with the patient; if you can, leave the situation and return later to let them cool off.
Sit down but, if you must stand, keep an open stance so you can quickly move away from the patient if necessary. Turn your body slightly away from the patient with your arms at the side; keep your hands open and maintain eye contact.
Do not hit, push, pull, or retaliate against a resident, even if provoked; it may be considered assault.
Do not ignore a problem; try to find the cause.
Try to distract the patient.

8. A. Gloves should be removed before recording a procedure.

9. A,D. The normal heart rate for a newborn is 120 bpm to 160 bpm.

10. C. Signs and symptoms of kidney stones include severe pain in the back and side below the ribs; pain in the lower abdomen, thigh, and urethra; nausea/vomiting; fever and chills; difficulty urinating; painful urination; cloudy or foul smelling urine; blood in urine; etc.

11. A, B. Peanut butter is too thick to feed someone with trouble swallowing.

12. A. When administering enemas, the patient should in a left Sim's position.

13. C. Residents must be given 30 days notice before being transferred or discharged.

14. B,C. Keep rooms uncluttered and tell patients about where furniture and other things are placed.
Maintain adequate lighting and to reduce glare, keep light sources behind the patient instead of behind you. Ensure that patients can locate and touch the light before leaving the room. Before entering a room, identify and announce your presence. Tell patients when you leave a room. Explain any unusual sounds in the room. Use the hands of the clock to tell patients about the location of food on the plate. Follow facility guidelines for removing, cleaning, and reinserting artificial eyes.

15. C. As a nursing assistant, you record inputs/outputs throughout the day and the input/output totals must be documented in the patient's medical records at the end of your shift.

16. B. Lower abdominal cramps are normal during breastfeeding.

17. C. According to HIPAA, you may only share patient information with those that directly care for the patient.

18. B. Pulse oximetry measures the oxygen concentration in the blood. A reading of 95 to 100% is normal.

19. A,B,C. All of the above, except IV fluids, should be included in a patient's intake records. A nurse is responsible for charting IV fluids.

20. C, D. When treating patients suffering from nausea and vomiting: provide frequent mouth care and offer ice chips if the patient can't keep anything down

21. A, D. Signs and symptoms of hypothyroidism include fatigue, weakness, weight gain, constipation, and intolerance to cold.

22. C. Signs and symptoms of a stroke include weakness/numbness in the face and/or limbs, particularly on only one side of the body; facial drooping or drooling; aphasia

(inability to speak); nausea/vomiting; lost or dimmed vision; loss of balance; severe headache with sudden onset.

23. B. Condom catheters are changed daily after perineal care.

24. B. Hearing is the last sense you lose.

25. D. Before giving a patient a bath, the first thing you should do is check the care plan to see if they are allowed to have a bath.

26. A. Straight catheters are used to empty the bladder and are then removed. Indwelling catheters (retention or Foley catheters) remain in the bladder, allowing for urine to constantly drain.

27. B. Apply tape to the top, middle, and bottom of a dressing, with the tape extending several inches beyond the side of the dressing. Do not encircle a body part with tape as that can cut off circulation if swelling occurs. Tape is removed by pulling it towards the wound.

28. B,C. When collecting a sputum specimen, the patient should rinse their mouth with water and cough deeply for the sputum. Antiseptics may kill microbes, affecting the results of the test. Most microbes live deep within the lungs.

29. A, D. When dressing or undressing patients, you should remove clothing from the weak/paralyzed limb last and clothe the weak/paralyzed limb first.

30. D. Frequent ostomy pouch changes can irritate the skin, so pouches are only changed every 2 to 7 days and when there is a leak.

31. B. Rehabilitation is care, provided by a physical therapist, to restore a patient to the highest level of functioning possible. Restorative care, often provided after rehabilitation, is ongoing and includes physical, emotional, and psychological care to help maintain a patient's functioning; CNAs provide restorative care.

32. B,C. Diabetic patients should have regularly scheduled meals and snacks to maintain a steady supply of glucose. Inspect the skin daily, especially the feet, for signs of pain or decreased sensations which indicate neuropathy, redness, or skin sores which may indicate poor circulation. Avoid pressure on feet.

33. A. During a seizure, lower a patient to the floor to prevent falls, place something soft under the patient's head to prevent the head from striking the floor, turn the patient in their side and make sure the head is turned to the side, do not put anything in the

patient's mouth, do not try to stop or control the patient's movements.

34. B. Rigor mortis is the stiffening of joints and muscles after death; the patient's body is put in normal alignment before rigor mortis sets in.

35. D. When using a glass thermometer, you should shake the thermometer until the substance is below the 94F mark.

36. C. Speech language pathology focuses on restoring a patient's ability to speak, chew, or swallow.

37. B. Glucometers are used to measure blood glucose levels. Normal levels are between 80 to 120 mg/dL. Hypoglycemia is when blood glucose levels are less than or equal to 60 mg/dL. Hyperglycemia is when blood glucose levels are greater than or equal to 120 mg/dL.

38. D. Shingles is viral disease characterized by itchy and painful skin rashes with blisters; it is most common in those over 50 years old. It is caused by the same virus as chickenpox and is contagious until the shingle lesions crust over. Shingles are treated with antiviral drugs and take 3 to 5 weeks to heal.

39. B, C. Always hold linen away from the your body; your clothing is considered dirty. Do not shake linens because that can spread microbes. Do not let linen touch the floor; linens that touch the floor need to be changed promptly. Fold contaminated side inward; put the soiled linen inside a plastic bag, tie the bag, and put the bag in the soiled linen area.

40. B. Do not place a wet cast on a hard surface or put pressure on a wet cast, it can misshapen the cast.

41. B. Occupational therapy is used to help a patient gain or maintain the skills needed for activities of daily living. It often focuses on improving fine motor skills used for eating with utensils, brushing the teeth, etc. Physical therapy often focuses on larger muscle functions.

42. C. This is an example of bargaining.

43. A. Turn the patient and the patient's head to the side so that excess fluid runs out of the mouth; this prevents the person from choking and aspiration.

44. A. People with hearing impairments find it more difficult to hear high pitch sounds, echos, hollow sounds, fast speech, speech with accents, and when there is background noise.

45. C. Hold the penis and clean from the tip down to the base of the penis, using circular motions.

46. A. Signs of impending death include Cheyne-Stokes respirations (rapid, irregular, and shallow breathing followed by decreased breathing and periods of no breathing); decreased blood pressure; rapid, weak pulse; cold and blue lips, hands, feets; decreased body movement, functions and awareness.

47. B,C,D. Hypoglycemia can occur when a patient takes too much insulin; takes insulin without eating a meal; or takes insulin and eats a meal, but increases physical activity. Hypoglycemic patients may exhibit bizarre and confused behavior. Other signs and symptoms include tachycardia; pale, cool skin; rapid, shallow breathing.

48. D. You must draw out all the water from the balloon; otherwise you can injured the urethra when removing the catheter. If there are 10 mL of water in the balloon and you were only able to draw out 9 mL, do not remove the catheter and immediately notify the nurse.

49. B. Patients should avoid food and fluids during surgery to reduce the risk of vomiting and aspirating the food/fluid.

50. C. When caring for patients with hip fractures, you should: prevent external rotation of the hip, keep the hip abducted and do not exercise the affected leg, do not let the person put weight on the affected leg unless ordered by a doctor, tell patients to not cross their legs, introduce weight bearing exercises to strengthen bones when appropriate as ordered by the care plan.

51. A. To relieve pain and swelling from a musculoskeletal injury, apply a cold compress.

52. D. Thrombosis is the formation of a clot in a blood vessel and is considered a medical emergency. Signs and symptoms include a red and warm area in the leg, pain which increases with movement, swelling, etc. Do not massage the leg, ambulate the patient, nor bend the toes upward as these actions can dislodge the clot and cause it to travel elsewhere. Report this to a licensed nurse immediately.

53. A, D. A person is only contagious when they have an active TB infection. Patients with TB can be treated in long term care facilities only if there are environmental controls in place and the facility has a respiratory protection program. Wear a TB respirator when treating a TB patient or entering the home or room of a TB patient. TB patients should wear masks when being transported, in waiting areas, and when others are present.

54. A, B. A nursing assistant's responsibility in rehabilitation and restorative care includes encouraging patients to practice techniques they've learned, reporting any observations

related to rehabilitation, and providing emotional support. It does not involve teaching patients techniques to regain function.

55. A,D. The average adults outputs 800 to 2000 mL of urine in a 24 hour period.

56. B,C,D. It is important that you treat patients with respect and care. To show your respect, call patients by their name and title instead of "Honey" or "Sweetie". Show care by spending time, showing interest, and listening to patients. Encourage social interactions and patient participation in their care to promote a sense of independence.

57. B. Delusions are false beliefs.

58. A.
First degree/superficial burns: affects the epidermis only; painful and red, but no blisters.
Second degree/partial thickness burns: affects the epidermis and parts of dermis, painful, red, and blisters.
Third degree/full thickness burns: affects entire dermis and there is no pain; skin may appear white and waxy or black and charred.

59. A. Signs and symptoms of an allergic reaction includes hives/rashes, tongue and facial swelling, wheezing or trouble breathing, vomiting/nausea, diarrhea.

60. C. Post surgery, have patients practice coughing and deep breathing exercise, and incentive spirometry to prevent respiratory complications such as pneumonia and atelectasis. To promote comfort, have patients hold a pillow or their hand over their incision site when coughing.

61. A. The catheter should be secured to the upper thigh. Taping the catheter to the outer thigh, bed, or knee can cause pulling/removal when a patient is turned.

62. B. Methicillin Resistant Staphylococcus Aureus (MRSA) is a bacterial infection of the skin that can spread to the bloodstream; it's especially prevalent in hospitals and long term care facilities.

63. D. Foods that are considered clear liquids include water, gelatin, fat-free broth, clear juices, clear carbonated sodas, and coffee and tea (without cream).

64. C. Canes should be held 6 to 10 inches to the side and 6 to 10 inches in front of the strong foot.

65. B. You should offer to contact a pastor or spiritual leader. Avoiding the topic and sharing your beliefs does not put the patient's needs first.

66. C. Always use electric razors for patients using anticoagulant drugs or patient's with blood clotting issues.

67. A. You should remain calm and comfort the patient. An anxious person will have a hard time calming themselves and you shouldn't try to distract them with more stimuli.

68. A,B,C,D. All of the above are benefits of bathing.

69. D. Hepatitis is a viral liver infection. Signs and symptoms include jaundice (yellowing of the skin or whites of the eyes), fatigue, loss of appetite, pain, nausea/vomiting, dark urine, skin rash, etc.

70. A. When performing abdominal thrusts, your fist should be placed above the patient's navel.

Thank You For Your Purchase

Thank you for your purchase. If you found this study guide helpful, please leave a review for us on Amazon; we would truly appreciate it.

If you have any questions or concerns, please contact us at goldstartestprep@gmail.com.

Bibliography

Sorrentino, Sheila A. and Leighann N. Remmert. Mosby's Textbook for Nursing Assistants 9th Edition. St. Louis, 2017.

Carter, Pamela J. Lippincott's Textbook for Nursing Assistants 4th Edition. China, 2016.

Whitenton, Linda and Marty Walker. Exam Cram Certified Nursing Assistant 2nd Edition. Indianapolis, 2017.

Pearson Vue. Skills Listing for the 2018 NNAAP. 2018.

Made in the USA
Columbia, SC
11 December 2019